Irritable Bowel Syndrome

Navigating Your Way to Recovery

Dr Megan Arroll

and

Professor Christine Dancey

With a Foreword by
Douglas A Drossman MD

and a Preamble by
Cecilia Håkanson, RN PhD

Hammersmith Health Books
London, UK

First published in 2016 by Hammersmith Health Books – an imprint
of Hammersmith Books Limited
4/4a Bloomsbury Square, London WC1A 2RP, UK
www.hammersmithbooks.co.uk

Disclaimer: The information contained in this book is for educational
purposes only. It is the result of the study and experience of the
authors. Whilst the information and advice offered are believed to be
true and accurate at the time of going to press, neither the authors nor
the publisher can accept any legal responsibility or liability for any
errors or omissions that may have been made or for any adverse effects
which may occur as a result of following the recommendations given
herein. Always consult a qualified medical practitioner if you have any
concerns regarding your health.

British Library Cataloguing in Publication Data: A CIP record of this
book is available from the British Library.

Print ISBN 978-1-78161-069-5
Ebook ISBN 978-1-78161-070-1

Commissioning editor: Georgina Bentliff
Designed by: Julie Bennett, Bespoke Publishing Ltd
Cover design and typesetting by: Sylvia Kwan
Index: Dr Laurence Errington
Production: Helen Whitehorn, Path Projects Ltd
Printed and bound by: TJ International Ltd

Contents

Acknowledgements

We would like to thank Professor Douglas Drossman for agreeing to read the manuscript and his kind input into the book in addition to writing the foreword despite his many other work commitments. We would also like to thank Dr Cecilia Håkanson for going through the draft manuscript and for making so many useful comments and suggestions for change. This has helped us enormously in improving the book. We thank Dr Håkanson also for contributing the book's Preamble.

We would like to thank Jo Johnstone, as always, for her expert proof-reading and feedback. We would also like to thank Maureen O'Hara and Matt Bowskill, who carefully read our manuscript and provided detailed feedback – the book has benefited greatly from their suggestions.

Finally, we would also like to thank all the people with IBS who kindly gave their time to share their personal experiences of IBS and who gave permission to use their narratives in the book.

Preface

Thirty years ago, in South London, Christine developed what appeared to be the symptoms of IBS – mostly abdominal pain, and bowel problems. She had various tests, including a barium enema and barium meal. The tests showed she did not have inflammatory bowel disease or cancer. As Christine at that time had no knowledge of endometriosis, she believed the doctors when they said she had irritable bowel syndrome (IBS). None of the medications prescribed improved Christine's symptoms; even when she had additional symptoms that were not consistent with IBS, various doctors maintained that she had IBS and that the additional symptoms were due to stress.

Christine felt let down by the health system and set about finding a self-help group to join. After searching extensively she didn't find any groups but she did find someone who was herself looking to find an IBS self-help group – Sue Backhouse, who lived in Sheffield. They began corresponding and decided to write a newsletter that they could send out to people with the condition and which hopefully would lead to setting up a self-help group. They contacted gastroenterologists and doctors and asked them to contribute. Christine telephoned a radio station and asked to be allowed to talk about IBS and encouraged anyone listening who had the symptoms to contact her for a newsletter. The newsletter, a simple two-sided document, was called *Gut Reaction* and their organisation, 'The IBS Network'. Around 50 people replied. More publicity, in magazines and newspapers, led to 10,000 letters in big sacks being delivered to Christine's house. It was obvious that there was a big need for information for people who had the symptoms of IBS. Friends and families rallied round to answer all the letters and it took many weeks to get the newsletters printed and sent out.

As a University lecturer and researcher, Christine then decided to do some research into the condition. She was amazed to find that there were hardly any papers or books for the layperson on IBS. There were medical papers but these were not written in a style that laypeople would find useful. Christine and Sue began to find out how people felt about their illness by asking people from the IBS Network how it affected their lives. Together they published an article and four books on the subject. Members of the IBS Network created more self-help groups and the newsletter, now a much improved glossy magazine (still called *Gut Reaction*) was read by around 12,000 in the UK. The IBS Network became a charity, with employees and volunteers. It was the only national organisation in the UK that helped people with IBS.

In 1992, after having a laparoscopy privately, Christine found out she had stage 4 endometriosis. Her bladder and bowel were attached to her womb by adhesions. As the endometriosis had not been caught in time, she was unable to have children. After hormone treatment she had a full hysterectomy. When she told her NHS doctors about this, they maintained that she had both IBS *and* endometriosis. Strangely, after correct treatment for endometriosis, Christine never again suffered from 'IBS symptoms'.

Christine continued to research into the causes and effects of IBS with other researchers in the UK, Europe and the USA. She also formed the Chronic Illness Research Team in her university and led that team until her retirement in 2012. Christine and Meg are both members of the team and continue to research into long-term conditions, including IBS.

Meg's personal interest in IBS stems from her having an over-lapping condition – myalgic encephalomyelitis, also known as chronic fatigue syndrome (ME/CFS). She was ill with glandular fever when she was 14 years old and went on to develop ME/CFS. She spent two years in bed and had to use home tutors to finish her GCSEs – her school was not helpful at all and insisted she was 'school phobic'. Doctors at the time were also pretty unhelpful, prescribing antidepressants and generally making the situation much, much worse.

After Meg finally had a diagnosis of ME from an educational psychologist, the family decided to take back control of Meg's health and used a pattern of rest and short bouts of activity (mainly school work). Although they did not know this at the time, in fact what Meg was doing was a form of what is now called 'pacing'. Very slowly she began to improve and was eventually able to go to university in London.

When Meg was trying to decide what to do for her PhD topic years later, she looked into what research was published on ME/CFS and was, like Christine and the topic of IBS, very surprised to see how little research had been published on the condition in comparison to other illnesses. So she carried out her PhD on ME/CFS and has been researching the illness since. Unfortunately, Meg too has had IBS on top (or as part) of the ME/CFS and was again shocked at what little help and information she received from her doctor.

When Meg joined the University of East London (UEL) as a lecturer it was clear that she and Christine had a great deal in common and that their previous work, looking at the patients' perspective in numerous illnesses, including IBS and ME/CFS, was similar. Between them, they have published almost 100 academic papers on IBS, ME/CFS, inflammatory bowel disease, Meniere's disease, *mal de debarquement* syndrome and other invisible, misunderstood and often stigmatised conditions. They are dedicated to carrying out research so that doctors, other researchers and the wider public can gain a greater understanding of what life is like for people with these long-term illnesses. They also collaborate with scientists from various disciplines, including immunology, cardiology and medical imaging, in their research studies. This, along with closely monitoring the scientific literature in the area of health, informs them of possible causes, underlying mechanisms and new treatments.

In this book, Meg and Christine have attempted to condense all the information that they have gathered on IBS into one publication, to make a comprehensive but accessible patient resource that is up to date and sorely needed in this area. Meg and Christine sincerely hope you will find the book useful and it will help you in your own personal journey.

Foreword

The understanding and care of persons with irritable bowel syndrome (IBS), the prototype of the functional gastrointestinal disorders (FGIDs), has long been challenging. Despite its high prevalence in the community and within clinical practice, knowledge of its pathophysiology has been limited, albeit growing, and when seeking diagnosis, we have come to realise that finding a single cause, or one specific treatment, is not only unlikely, but is based on false assumptions.

IBS is truly a biopsychosocial disorder; the causes are multi-determined, and vary depending on the individual's genetic make-up, microenvironment, psychological state, and the foods eaten. To truly understand IBS one must appreciate the immense variability in symptoms and their severity across persons so afflicted and in the same person over time. So, while having IBS means fulfilling certain symptom (Rome) criteria (see page 11), the clinical expression of this disorder and the personal experience of having it can vary considerably and be truly unique to the individual. Thus, having IBS can be confusing to persons so afflicted and even to the clinicians caring for them.

Through my research and clinical care of patients coming to me for decades and my role as President of the Rome Foundation, I and other academics in the field have sought to teach the diagnosis and care of persons with IBS to scientists and clinicians. But as it is said 'it takes two to tango', so persons so afflicted must also understand their disorder in order to engage effectively with their clinicians and participate in their care, including self-management. Knowledge is indeed power.

Dr Megan Arroll and Professor Christine Dancey have now created remarkable guidance to help persons with IBS in their journey of understanding and self-management of their disorder. In their new book, *Irritable Bowel Syndrome: Navigating your way to recovery*, they begin with an overview of IBS that covers the symptoms, pathophysiological features and diagnosis, and introduce the concept of the brain-gut axis, which is so important to achieving a full understanding. They then cover such important topics as explanatory models of IBS, diagnosis using the Rome criteria, and medical, nutritional and psychological treatments. Great emphasis is placed on techniques for self-management and the book even ends with a guide for family, friends and colleagues.

The book is fresh and up to date. To begin with they move away from IBS being called a 'functional' gastrointestinal disorder. Although 'functional' means disorder of gut function, most of the general public and even clinicians interpret the term as implying psychological, unknown or 'the absence of real disease' and these erroneous definitions can lead to frustration, stigmatisation and the application of unneeded diagnostic studies and treatments. Indeed, the Rome Foundation which provides guidance to practitioners in the field has renamed functional GI disorders as 'Disorders of gut–brain interaction' that result from any combination of: 1) disturbed motility (movement of the intestine), 2) visceral hypersensitivity (increased pain from the intestinal nerves), 3) altered mucosal and immune function of the bowel, and 4) altered gut microbiota (composition of bacteria in the gut) and altered central nervous system processing of gut function (the brain–gut axis). Indeed, Dr Arroll and Professor Dancey cover all these topics in their book in a concise and easy-to-understand way.

There are several features that make this book particularly helpful for those seeking to understand and manage their IBS. The first is the discussion of the intestinal microenvironment: the microbiome, gut permeability, immune dysfunction and the role of bacteria provide a concise view of one of the key features of IBS pathogenesis. This understanding can help to explain why treatments like probiotics can be helpful. Second, the discussion of the role of stress in this disorder is very well handled and is non-stigmatising. From its embryonic beginnings, the brain and gut have been 'hardwired' to each other and this explains why stress can affect intestinal function, intestinal pain can lead to greater anxiety and even psychiatric treatments can also help the gut. Third, the discussion of the diagnostic studies that physicians may consider in the evaluation is complete and easy to follow. Fourth, I like the idea of using quotes from persons with IBS in order to help others know that they are not alone in their thoughts and feelings. Fifth, there is an excellent discussion on the role of the family, who we know also share the experience of the illness with their loved ones. Finally I very much like the emphasis in this book on what people can do to get relief. It can be empowering to acquire personal resources and self-manage.

As the field of medicine moves towards a more integrated, biopsychosocial understanding of illness and disease, and towards a patient-centred plan of care, persons with IBS and other functional GI disorders are likely to benefit. This book I believe will help us to move in that direction. I highly recommend this book for anyone with IBS, or who has a family member or friend with IBS or who cares for those with IBS.

Douglas A Drossman MD
President, Rome Foundation
Professor Emeritus of Medicine and Psychiatry, University of North Carolina at Chapel Hill, US
President, Center for Education and Practice of Biopsychosocial Care LLC
Drossman Gastroenterology PLLC

Preamble

Irritable bowel syndrome (IBS) is an invisible, fluctuating disease and as such it is often difficult for family members, friends, colleagues, health service professionals, welfare insurance administrators and others who encounter people with the disease to understand the suffering of the individual.

People with IBS are often faced with troublesome and sometimes severe physical symptoms that in different ways obstruct or challenge their everyday life. The disease is by its nature potentially shameful. In our modern western society some of our most fundamental bodily functions, like flatulence and defecation, are considered to be private and nothing you would want others to know about. Hence, for many persons with IBS, sharing their illness experience does not come easily.

Among healthcare professionals, knowledge about IBS is quite often insufficient and it is regarded as a low-priority disease. Sometimes IBS patients find that their troubles are dismissed or belittled, for example, in healthcare encounters or by family members. Not being taken seriously – at home or by healthcare professionals – can be a devastating experience which affects self-image. For some people getting the diagnosis is affirming, providing a legitimate passport to the healthcare system. For others, however, being diagnosed means nothing but being a 'closed case', and they feel left with insufficient information, advice and support. They find they have more questions than answers. In the jungle of potential self-management suggestions (available through various websites, blogs and chat forums) about what to eat, when to sleep or how to behave if you get urgent bowel movements and start to panic on the bus, it is easy to get confused. Being on your own, having to figure out how to live the rest of your life with an illness that won't go away, and a disease for which there is no treatment or clear and certain 'rules' to follow but learning to know one's own body and what works best, is not an easy task.

Literature about IBS has until now tended to be either too medically oriented, complex and difficult for lay people to understand, or to be like a pamphlet, too brief to be useful. This book is therefore a very much welcomed contribution for all laypersons – people with IBS, family members, colleagues, neighbours and others who for some reason need to learn more about the disease, what life with IBS is about and what help is out there. The book offers a thorough explanation of the mechanisms and (as far as there is scientific evidence) likely causes of IBS, and of available pharmacological and non-pharmacological treatment options. It also portrays life with the illness from the perspective of those who live with the disease, and linked to this, a variety of self-care strategies are described. The book can of course be read as a whole, but it also forms a very useful reference book for certain aspects or topics of particular interest to the reader. I am certain that anyone who is interested in knowing more, or has specific questions, about IBS will find useful information and answers to their questions.

Cecilia Håkanson RN, PhD
Researcher and Senior Lecturer
Ersta Sköndal University College, Stockholm, Sweden

Cecilia Håkanson RN, PhD is a researcher and senior lecturer at the Palliative Research Centre and the Department of Health Care Sciences at Ersta Sköndal University College, Stockholm, Sweden. She is also an affiliated researcher at Karolinska Institutet, Department of Neurobiology, Care Science and Society, in Stockholm, Sweden.

Cecilia has a background in nursing, with many years of clinical experience of IBS. She gained her PhD in 2010, based on a thesis project about everyday life, healthcare encounters and patient education among people with IBS. Her post-doctoral studies have mainly been performed in the field of life-limiting illness, dying and palliative care, concerning aspects of bodily experiences, bodily care and person centredness, and place of care and death with focus on aspects of quality and equality. She has also performed research about eating difficulties at the end of life, and about providing and receiving care in the context of being homeless and severely ill.

About the authors

Dr Megan Arroll PhD, CPsychol, CSci, FHEA, AFBPsS, is a psychologist and health researcher who specialises in stress and anxiety, invisible/misunderstood illness and integrative approaches to healthcare. Megan has held academic positions at a number of universities and lectures on a range of topics, including mental health, the psychology of health & illness and research methods. Over recent years Megan has been writing books for patients, their families and people working with long-term conditions. To date she has published four books including *Chronic Fatigue Syndrome: What You Need to Know About CFS/ME* (SPCK) and *The Menopause Maze: The Complete Guide to Conventional, Complementary and Self-Help Options* (Singing Dragon) with Liz Efiong.

Professor Christine Dancey PhD, CPsychol, CHealth Psychol, FHEA, FBPsS, is Professor Emeritus of Chronic Illness Research at the University of East London (UEL) and best-selling author. Her numerous titles include *Statistics Without Maths for Psychology* (Pearson) which has been used to help many thousands of students understand the complex mathematics involved in scientific research. Christine was also the joint founder of the IBS Network and its publication *Gut Reaction* (www.theibsnetwork. org/gut-reaction/), which is now available as an online download for members. As a researcher into invisible long-term conditions and a misdiagnosed sufferer from IBS symptoms, she has a unique insight into what people with IBS and their families and friends want and need to know.

Megan met Christine at the University of East London, where Christine led the Chronic Illness Research Team. Within this research group, Megan and Christine published numerous papers on long-term conditions, such as CFS/ME, Ménière's disease and irritable bowel syndrome (IBS). When the pair's students started to ask for easy-to-read books about some of these illnesses, Megan and Christine decided to start writing for the general public. Their first title was *Invisible Illness: Coping with Misunderstood Conditions* (SPCK), followed by *Irritable Bowel Syndrome: Navigating Your Way to Recovery* (Hammersmith Health Books). They are now working on their third book together, (*What's Up with Your Bladder?*) to be published in January 2018 (Hammersmith Health Books). These books include the very latest scientific research to keep patients up-to-date with developments in treatments and potential causes of ill health, in addition to practical advice on how to manage symptoms. Megan and Christine shared personal experience of invisible illness has given them not only the basis for a fulfilling writing partnership, but also a deep friendship.

How to use this book

In *Irritable Bowel Syndrome: Navigating your way to recovery*, we have tried to cover as many relevant topics as possible, but invariably there will be something that we have overlooked. Our aim was to write a practical self-help book to give enough information and advice to enable people to find strategies to deal with IBS; hence most of the chapters are about different treatments and techniques for managing and treating IBS symptoms. Chapter 1 includes a lot of detail on diagnosis so that prospective patients can know what to expect (or what they *should* expect) when visiting the doctor. However, even if you have a diagnosis already we do recommend that you start by reading this chapter as it gives some background and context to the illness. If you want to skip Chapter 1, Chapters 2–7 are stand-alone and you can flip from one to another as you wish.

Chapters 8 and 9 are much more technical as we wanted to outline the possible causes of IBS, old and new theories on how IBS develops (known as explanatory models), and current research that is leading researchers and doctors to a better understanding of what is going on in the bodies of individuals with IBS. We have endeavoured to simplify the more technical information and put it together in a sensible way, but you may not be interested in this more in-depth research. This is okay too as not knowing all the details of recent research won't prevent patients from being able to access the treatments and support they may need to start getting their lives back on track.

Finally, we end with a separate section for relatives and friends, which we hope will enable them to better support the person with IBS and help them regain good health. They can be asked to read just this chapter – they needn't read the entire book in order to give the care and understanding required to tackle this condition.

We sincerely hope you find this book helpful.
Megan and Christine

Chapter 1

Introduction to IBS

'The pathogenesis of IBS appears to be multifactorial. The following play a central role in the pathogenesis: heritability and genetics, dietary and intestinal microbiota, low-grade inflammation and disturbances in the neuroendocrine system of the gut.'

Khanbhai and Sura[1]

This chapter introduces the most recent research into an extremely common condition from which you, or someone known to you, may be suffering – irritable bowel syndrome or IBS. A lot of the research is very medically based and incredibly complex. To write an accessible book that is informative and understandable, we have simplified some of the more complex ideas. A number of the terms medical scientists use will be unfamiliar to some readers – for instance, the quote above, written for an academic medical audience, means:

'The origin and development of IBS appears to have many causes. The following factors have a central role in the causes and development of the condition: genetics – a certain likelihood of developing IBS could be inherited; types of foods eaten and the trillions of micro-organisms (gut flora, or 'microbiota') that live in the gut; low-level inflammation in the gut; the communication between the brain and gut might be disturbed.'

In taking a complex quote and re-phrasing it so that non-academic, non-medical people can understand it, we hope that we have done justice to the original. However, often when people simplify things, they lose some of the accuracy and meaning that the original authors and medical academics intended. Obviously we have tried not to lose any accuracy but we have also included the related references so that you can look at the original research papers for yourself should you so wish.

In this chapter we give a brief overview of IBS, which includes general information about the ways in which it is viewed by health professionals, academics and everyone working in the area of gastroenterology. We give more specific information about the economic and social costs of IBS and its symptoms and provide information on the prevalence of the condition (that is the number of people who currently have the disease). We have included information relating to the diagnostic criteria used to determine whether a person is likely to have IBS and information on other diseases that it may be mistaken for. Diagnostic tests are discussed in Chapter 3 (pages 38–47).

In the chapters that follow we will illustrate the relationship between the brain and the gut, and introduce the work that shows how the resident bacteria in the gut play a larger part in the development of the disease than was previously thought and what the implications are for treatment.

Diagnosing IBS

Symptoms

The following are some of the very unpleasant symptoms of IBS. The frequency, severity, and type may differ between different people and can vary within an individual on a day-to-day or month-to-month basis:

1   **Abdominal pain** – This can be anywhere between mild to extremely severe, related to bowel movements and, for women, can vary with the menstrual cycle.

2   **A change of bowel habits** – People vary a lot in their bowel movements. It is a *change* in bowel habit that is important here. Someone who has always had to battle with constipation may start to get diarrhoea, or someone used to loose bowel movements may suddenly become constipated. Any change in bowel habit needs checking out.

3   **Urgency to have a bowel movement** – This affects people with both diarrhoea and constipation and those who alternate between the two. This is a very difficult symptom to deal with since bowel incontinence can result if the individual cannot get to a toilet quickly. This, needless to say, can be both embarrassing and upsetting.

4   **'Burbulence'** – People who have IBS often find they have rumblings and grumblings in the digestive system; this is called 'burbulence'.

5   **Flatulence, wind, and bloating** are also common.

You may have heard the abbreviations IBS-C and IBS-D; these are used because most people tend to have IBS with predominant constipation (IBS-C) or diarrhoea (IBS-D). However, as mentioned, these patterns can change and patients can go from feeling completely bunged up to rushing for the toilet to prevent an accident. In Chapter 3 we will discuss how symptoms can be tracked in order to find out if there are any identifiable reasons for changes in the symptom patterns being experienced.

Prevalence

It is estimated that in western society, around 20% of women, and

10% of men, have symptoms of IBS. In the UK it is estimated that the prevalence is 17% overall (11% of men and 23% of women).

Many people who have symptoms of IBS do not consult a healthcare professional, hence the prevalence of the illness in the general population is likely to be higher than the number of those actually diagnosed.

As the figures above imply, women are twice as likely to have symptoms of IBS as men and, as would be expected, the rates of diagnosis are higher as well. Thus, IBS has been traditionally seen as a women's illness. Recently researchers looking at the nerve cells that control the movement of food through the digestive system have shown differences between men and women which could go some way to explaining why this is[2]. However, more women than men consult their GP about their symptoms, so it may be that men simply suffer in silence a lot of the time.

A diagnosis of IBS has been (and is currently) made on the basis of the symptoms themselves and in the absence of any other disease process that could account for the symptoms. In addition, there are no standard biomarkers for IBS *as yet*. This means that there are no standard laboratory tests that can tell whether or not someone has IBS; the test results will come up as 'normal'. If they are not normal, then it is likely that the patient will have further tests to determine which of a number of conditions he/she may have. The tests a person is likely to have in order to rule out other diseases are discussed in Chapter 3.

Social costs of IBS

IBS intrudes into the lives of millions of people and can be a big challenge to anyone who is trying to cope with the illness, especially at times when other people are less than supportive. Luckily, most people have heard about IBS and know other people who have the symptoms, so understanding is generally greater than it was 30 years ago; this makes a huge difference to people with a long-term condition such as this. We know that traditionally IBS has been stigmatised – that is, people with the condition have felt ashamed of having it because of the attitudes of others. People used to laugh when IBS was mentioned and even health professionals such as nurses believed these patients were malingerers and were wasting doctors' time! If you read the first books on IBS by Christine Dancey and Sue Backhouse[3,4] you will see just how negative attitudes were in those days. (These books are very out of date now so we don't recommend them for information about IBS).

Many people used to believe that IBS was a psychosomatic disorder. 'Psychosomatic', in the true sense of the word, means that psychological factors express themselves in bodily symptoms. This means that stress, anxiety or depression may express themselves as IBS, myalgic encephalomyelitis/chronic fatigue syndrome (ME/CFS), or any other type of invisible illness. As we have shown in our previous books, it is possible that stress in particular plays a part in all illnesses. However, as in other chronic illnesses, IBS is not 'all in the mind'. In fact, people who think IBS is a psychosomatic disorder are now in the minority. Even 10 years ago, the vast majority of consultant doctors (80%) believed that IBS was a medical disorder – but that the medical explanation just hadn't been found yet. Now, it seems certain that IBS, like other chronic disorders, is a result of interactions between different factors. Stress can trigger IBS – but not in the simplistic way that many people believe. It can do so through neuro-psycho-physio-somatic mechanisms. This means that it is the interaction between neurological (brain and nervous system), psychological, physiological and biological factors.

For example, there may be a genetic predisposition to IBS as it has been shown that genetics do play a part in IBS (see Chapter 8). Also, gut microbiota are very important in health and illness (see also Chapter 9). Acute early stress may sensitise the gut so that later stress has a bigger impact on it than in people who did not experience the acute early stress (see Chapter 9). The gut may also have been rendered more permeable ('leaky'), which some experts think may contribute to IBS. So, neurological, psychological and physiological factors together can lead to conditions such as IBS and other medically unexplained conditions, such as ME/CFS and fibromyalgia. If we can discover the ways in which these factors interact to trigger IBS, then it is entirely possible that new treatments could make life bearable again. (Life with IBS is discussed more fully in Chapter 2.)

Economic costs of IBS

People with IBS use 50% more healthcare resources than people who do not have IBS. All illnesses and diseases have economic costs, to the healthcare system, employers, and the individual concerned. These costs include the number of days of work missed due to illness, loss of productivity at work, prescription costs and the costs of repeated visits to the GP or hospital. Around 20% of people diagnosed with IBS undergo medical procedures such as colonoscopy, endoscopy, and sigmoidoscopy (described in Chapter 3).

The total financial burden attributable to IBS is similar to that of other long-term illnesses such as asthma. One French study found that most prescriptions were given for abdominal pain and bloating and that around 8% of patients had been hospitalised due to IBS during the preceding year[5]. The average total annual direct cost per patient was €756 (about £600).

As so many people have IBS, finding effective treatments – or even a total cure – should be a top priority for healthcare professionals, even without considering the economic costs, which should be an additional incentive.

Other diseases with symptoms in common with IBS

It is important to know about other diseases that have sometimes been mistaken for IBS. In such cases, people have the symptoms of IBS but may also have additional symptoms that are not consistent with the condition. Sometimes people do not mention these additional symptoms to their doctor, possibly because of embarrassment. Sometimes the additional symptoms occur after a person has been given a diagnosis of IBS, in which case they should go back to their GP.

IBS has sometimes been diagnosed when the person concerned has had the following conditions.

Inflammatory bowel disease (IBD)

IBD consists of two diseases: Crohn's disease and ulcerative colitis. Both of these related diseases show a clear disease process upon testing. Symptoms include diarrhoea and abdominal pain, in common with IBS, and also fatigue. However, there are a range of laboratory tests that can show whether IBD is present (see Chapter 3). Despite this, a recent study found that around 10% of IBD patients were misdiagnosed with IBS and for 3% of those patients the misdiagnosis lasted for five or more years[6].

Coeliac disease

Symptoms in common with IBS are diarrhoea and/or constipation, abdominal pain, bloating and fatigue.

People who have this disease are allergic to gluten, which occurs in grains such as wheat, barley and rye, and is in many grain-based foods, such as bread, pasta, biscuits and cereals. Coeliac disease is an auto-immune condtion in which the body perceives the gluten to be a threat and therefore produces antibodies against it, causing inflammation in the intestines. Blood tests and a biopsy of the gut can confirm whether or not someone has coeliac disease.

Lactose intolerance

Some people are intolerant of milk and milk products because they do not produce enough of an enzyme called lactase which is responsible for the digestion of the sugar in milk – lactose. This deficiency can lead to symptoms similar to IBS – those include, abdominal pain, bloating and diarrhoea. An elimination diet, hydrogen breath test and testing a sample of faeces can indicate whether or not a person is intolerant of lactose.

Endometriosis

Endometriosis is a gynaecological disease in which cells from the womb migrate to other sites in the body, bleed with the monthly menstrual cycle and become infected. Adhesions may bind parts of the bowel or bladder to the womb. This can lead to abdominal pain, fatigue and difficulty (with pain) when having a bowel movement. There are other symptoms that endometriosis does not have in common with IBS, including painful and/or heavy periods and a muddy discharge in between periods.

Research has shown that 7% of women who were finally diagnosed with endometriosis were previously diagnosed with IBS. Most found their 'IBS' was no longer present after successful treatment for endometriosis. Unfortunately it takes an average of 7.5 years between a woman first seeing a GP about her symptoms and receiving a firm diagnosis of endometriosis.

IBS – cause or causes?

Most IBS books written for the layperson list the possible causes of IBS (for instance, diet, stress, anxiety), as if they are mutually exclusive. IBS and other medically unexplained disorders, such as ME/CFS and fibromyalgia, are rarely due to one cause. Most of these conditions are now believed to be multi-causal, that is, the causes interact together to trigger symptoms, usually in someone predisposed to the illness. Remember the quote at the beginning of this chapter? That came from a highly respected journal called the *Journal of Medical Practitioners*. The authors were describing IBS as having several causes. These could be genetic – relatives of someone with IBS are two to three times as likely to have IBS as someone with no family history of the condition. Dietary factors (including intestinal microbiota), low-grade inflammation and disturbances in the hormonal system of the gut also play a central part. A bout of gastroenteritis can also trigger IBS (see Chapter 9). Needless to say, experts who have studied gastroenterology have different perspectives on IBS, often disagreeing with each other as to the relative importance of the cause or causes of IBS. They also have different views on how IBS should be treated. After all, if someone thinks IBS is due to stress, they would treat it very differently from someone who believes it is due to low-grade inflammation. Most experts, however, as we have said, believe that IBS has more than one cause.

In addition, although people talk about 'psychological' and 'physical' illness, we have shown previously that the body/brain/mind are not separate entities (see, for example, *Invisible Illness: Coping with Misunderstood Conditions*[7]. All the bodily systems and brain systems are involved both in health and in illness. Bodily systems, such as the nervous system, hormones, digestive, respiratory, cardiovascular and immune systems, all communicate with each other and physical factors, such as infections and allergies, and psychosocial factors, such as stress, can together trigger an immune response in the body that increases its susceptibility to illness.

People of course have different views or perspectives about IBS (and other illnesses). These are called 'models'. A common model of IBS, for instance, is the 'biopsychosocial model' where it is believed that IBS is the result of several factors interacting together: biological, psychological, and social. Recently, some researchers have questioned this view, believing that medical factors will explain IBS without recourse to psychological and social factors; this would be a 'medical model'.

You too will have particular views about IBS. Your view/model of IBS may differ from that of your GP. We carried out some research where we found that people who had similar views to their GP about the causes of IBS were happier with their doctor than those who saw things differently[8].

The causes and further models of IBS will be discussed in detail in Chapters 8 and 9. We will also include comparisons between GPs' and patients' perspectives and explanatory models and discuss the mismatch between the two.

Diagnostic criteria

There are specific criteria that health professionals use to diagnose IBS. Before these criteria were devised, IBS was known as 'spastic colon' or 'irritable colon syndrome' as symptoms were thought to be due entirely to gut spasms. Up until recently IBS has been thought of as purely a 'functional' disorder. This really means that no medical reason could be found for the condition. A common explanation given for the symptoms was some sort of life stress, but then there has always been a tendency, when no medical reasons can be found for a condition, to ascribe the problem to 'psychological factors'.

In the 1970s, researcher A P Manning and colleagues devised a set of criteria which could differentiate between those who had IBS and those who had an organic (medical) gut disease such as IBD. The first criteria were therefore called the Manning Criteria. Doctors and consultants were supposed to use these criteria to diagnose patients presenting with matching symptoms. However, some studies found that only around a quarter of GPs used them[9].

There then followed other, updated criteria, called the Rome criteria. These criteria were devised by international experts of gastroenterology who met in Rome in 1989 to develop and refine the criteria for IBS and other gastroenterological diseases. The first set of criteria were called the Rome I criteria, and these were followed by the Rome II and III criteria. The latter were devised in 2006 and are still in use today[10]. However, the different criteria have different sensitivity rates in diagnosing IBS. (Sensitivity means the ability of the criteria to correctly identify those who really have IBS and those who don't.) If different sets of criteria have different sensitivities you might find that an individual could be diagnosed as having IBS with one set of criteria, but not with the other. This is important, of course, because misdiagnosis is more likely to occur when the diagnostic criteria are not accurate. As other diseases have symptoms in common with IBS (such as IBD), it is very difficult to make a positive diagnosis of IBS without carrying out tests to exclude other conditions (these tests will be discussed in Chapter 3).

The following are the Rome III criteria for the diagnosis of irritable bowel syndrome. There must be:

A. Recurrent abdominal pain or discomfort (not actual pain) for the last three months, with the onset of symptoms being present for at least six months prior to diagnosis.

B. For at least three days a month in the last three months the patient must have experienced at least two of the following:

1. Improvement of abdominal pain or discomfort upon having a bowel movement

2. Onset associated with a change in frequency of stool

3. Onset associated with a change in form (appearance) of stool.

Rome IV criteria will be published in Spring 2016. Professor Douglas Drossman, writing about the new criteria, states:

> 'We also expect to show with Rome IV that we can finally discard the functional-organic dichotomy that tends to stigmatize these disorders. Functional GI disorders are now understood as having structural abnormalities in mucosal immune dysfunction and the microbiota and the work in biomarkers is likely to be a feature for understanding these disorders in the future.'
>
> *Professor Douglas Drossman*

This means that Professor Drossman doesn't believe we should label IBS as 'functional'. Functional disorders were often stigmatised because people knew that 'functional' meant there was no medical explanation for them. It's only a short step from this to thinking that if no cause could be found then perhaps there was 'nothing to be found'. The 'functional' label resulted in people with these conditions feeling stigmatised and as if the illness was their own fault. However, as we now know, with more research and hence more knowledge, there really is something wrong. Perhaps all functional disorders may in time be found to have a medical basis.

The gut and its relationship with the brain

The gut is a hollow flexible tube, approximately nine meters long, though the tube is folded up as you can see from Figure 1. The various muscles of the gut shorten and lengthen in order to squeeze the food along the digestive system, a process known as peristalsis. The workings of the gut are controlled by a system known as the enteric nervous system (ENS), which is located in the gut wall, so the gut effectively has its own 'nervous system'. We hardly notice the workings of our gut until something goes wrong. When everything works properly, food is moved along the gut until we have an easy bowel movement. However, we know that for millions of people worldwide, this isn't the case. For instance, they might experience a change from normal bowel habits to either diarrhoea or constipation, as well as having symptoms such as abdominal pain and bloating.

The system controlling the gut is called the brain–gut axis (BGA). The BGA includes the central nervous system (CNS), which consists of the brain and spinal cord, the enteric nervous system (in the gut), and the hypothalamic–pituitary–adrenal system or 'axis' (the HPA). These are briefly described below.

As we have pointed out, experts believe that stress aggravates any illness and is a factor in all illnesses. This is *not* simply a psychological phenomenon; things are far more complicated than that. Our bodies deal with stressful events by altering our physiology. You no doubt know about the 'fight or flight' mechanism. Faced with sudden, acute stress, our bodies act seemingly without our minds being involved. This is part of the CNS working really fast. Imagine you are walking home alone, on a dark night. No one seems to be around, but you can hear footsteps coming from somewhere. You begin to feel nervous. Your heartrate speeds up, and you are aware that someone is running to catch you up. Someone is about to attack you! Immediately your body prepares for this emergency. The hormones adrenaline and noradrenaline are released by the adrenal glands. After the CNS has begun working, the HPA axis starts a process which secretes a hormone called cortisol. Cortisol mobilises resources within the body to provide additional energy. It also aids regulation of the immune and cardiac systems. You will feel the effects of these

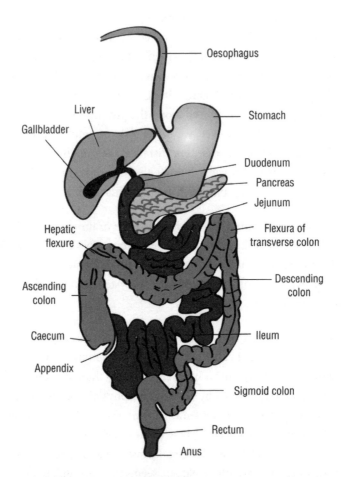

Figure 1 The gut – The oesophagus, stomach and small bowel (duodenum, jejunum and ileum) form the upper gut, and the colon and rectum form the large bowel/lower gut. All parts can be affected by IBS

changes in your body as blood pumps around your body faster and you can run more quickly.

Imagine now that you made a mistake; the person running is just a night-jogger, who jogs away in a different direction. How do you feel now? Probably it will take you some time to calm down as the hormones will still be racing through your body. Short, acute stress is dealt with by the nervous system, and when the threat is over, usually you just go back to your normal level of calmness.

The fast response by the CNS is followed by the slower-activating HPA axis. The hypothalamus communicates via nerves in the body with the nervous and endocrine systems through the pituitary and adrenal glands. It also communicates with the gut! If there is continued stress, the HPA system will continue to be activated, and various hormones will be released into the bloodstream. Examples of continuing stress might be the threat of redundancy hanging over you, or financial or relationship worries. Such continuing stress has subsequent effects on your body, and over time the HPA may not be able to regulate itself so well. The HPA system gives rise to an inflammatory response, which may be relevant for people with IBD and IBS. This is because even though the inflammatory response is our body's way of dealing with any threats (such as viruses, 'bad' bacteria, and fungi) and gives rise to the healing process, long-term inflammation can actually cause us damage. In the case of IBD and IBS, this damage is within the intestinal wall, leading to symptoms such as pain and diarrhoea. We will be talking more about the BGA/ HPA axis throughout the book. These systems are incredibly complex and a small book like this cannot possibly tell you all you might want to know about them. Recommendations are included in the Reference list on pages 162–8

Brain–gut interactions

The brain controls and governs our digestive system but the gut and the brain have two-way connections between them. These connections are made via neurotransmitters – chemicals that carry nerve signals across the central nervous system. When we talk about brain-gut interactions, we often call the actual brain 'the big brain' and the enteric nervous system (ENS) 'the small brain'. It is important to remember that the CNS, ENS and the HPA constitute the brain–gut axis (BGA). The BGA is involved in keeping balance and stability in the digestive system, appetite and weight control. The big brain is of course the most important organ in these processes.

Gut microbiota

Professor Douglas Drossman, an expert in IBS and IBD who has worked in gastroenterology for many decades, has stated that disorders such as IBS are due to 'mucosal immune dysfunction' and abnormalities in gut microbiota. The intestinal mucosa is the permeable lining of the gut which creates a barrier between internal and external environments. So, for instance, water will pass through the barrier, but pathogens (substances which cause disease) normally will not be able to pass through. This will be discussed further in Chapter 9.

In relation to gut microbiota, all of us have trillions of microorganisms (viruses, bacteria, fungi) in our body and most of these live on the inner surfaces of our intestines – these are what we call 'gut microbiota'. Gut microbiota have evolved to live with us in our body and are good for us. There is recent research showing that the gut microbiota play a much larger part in general health – and gut health in particular – than previously thought [11]. The gut microbiota enable all sorts of things to happen in the gut – they make sure that the mucosa works properly, they contribute to normal gut motility, so that the food passes through the system normally, that is not too fast and not too slow, and they also ensure that nutrients taken in when you eat are absorbed properly. They are also involved in the immune system and inflammatory responses. However, the gut microbiota can be disturbed by antibiotics, laxatives and other medications and by alterations within the gastrointestinal system. If the relationship between the microbiota and the big and little brain is disturbed (called dysbiosis), then diseases such as IBD and IBS can result. It is therefore possible that gastrointestinal diseases such as IBD and IBS might be helped by changing the gut microbiota.

If anyone tells you that IBS is simply due to stress or diet, you can tell them that this is a *very* simplistic view! Gut microbiota and the possible causes or triggers of IBS are discussed in detail in Chapter 9 (page 135).

Summary

In this chapter we have given a brief introduction to the topics that we will cover in this book. We have explained some key facts about IBS and introduced some important concepts, such as the brain-gut axis, the HPA axis, models of IBS and gut microbiota.

In the following chapters we will expand on these areas, discussing additional topics, such as diagnostic procedures, nutrition and treatments for IBS, and provide a guide for friends and family.

Chapter 2

Living and managing life with IBS

'A predominant theme [in a study of IBS patients] was a sense of stigma experienced because of a lack of understanding by family, friends and physicians of the effects of IBS on the individual, or the legitimacy of the individual's emotions and adaptation behaviors experienced. Patients described IBS not only as symptoms (predominantly abdominal pain) but mainly as it affects daily function, thoughts, feelings and behaviors. Common responses included uncertainty and unpredictability with loss of freedom, spontaneity and social contacts, as well as feelings of fearfulness.'

Drossman and colleagues[12]

In this chapter we look at what life is like for people with IBS, the difficulties they might be facing and how such problems contribute to a reduced quality of life. Having one thing that makes life difficult might not be too bad, but to have to face multiple difficulties can be very challenging indeed. We also offer advice on what can be done to better manage life with IBS.

'IBS and its symptoms are not a triviality or a figment of one's imagination – the pain is really debilitating, and not something

I wish for, or knowingly bring on. It just happens!'

Maria

How do we know what it's like to have IBS? Until the 1990s, we didn't know much. Books written on the subject tended to be for people who were medically trained, and apart from a book and a few small leaflets there was no detailed advice on how to cope with the condition and no information on patient perspectives in publications relating to IBS. There were no known self-help groups and most people had to cope the best they could with this limited information.

Now we have many books on the subject and studies that look at the views of people with IBS themselves. We know how much IBS affects people's lives and the ways in which they cope. There are studies that analyse the ways that patients make sense of their disease, the ways their lives are affected and the problems they have with healthcare professionals, friends, families and workmates.

People with IBS have to cope with painful, unpredictable and embarrassing symptoms. These symptoms are largely hidden from others, except when they are told about them. Research studies show that IBS leads to a worsening of quality of life, problems with relationships and feelings of shame and stigma. However, most people with IBS are coping well with a disease that is still misunderstood by many people.

What makes life difficult for people with IBS?

Unpredictability

IBS, ME/CFS, inflammatory bowel disease, Meniere's disease and any disorders or conditions that have unpredictable symptoms make day-to-day living difficult. One study carried out by a Norwegian team led by Professor Marit Rønnevig looked at the experiences of people living with IBS[13]. The team carried out open-ended interviews and the top theme that emerged from people's accounts was 'living with unpredictability'. People with IBS felt out of control, constrained and dependent. Other studies also showed that the symptoms of IBS affect daily life, with unpredictability and uncertainty being a big problem. In Chapter 7 (page 107) we'll explore some strategies that can help with this unpredictability and any sudden attacks of IBS symptoms.

A particular problem for the people in the above study was the unpredictability of symptoms such as diarrhoea or urgency when out of the house. Sometimes the symptoms came on really suddenly and then they had to find a toilet very quickly; what they feared most was not reaching a toilet in time.

> 'The IBS affects so many parts of my life: family occasions and my enjoyment of them, holidays when I am in pain, and my intimate relationship, as I experience discomfort sometimes during intimacy. When my IBS is playing up, all I want to do is curl up on my bed/sofa, with a heat pad on my stomach. I lose my energy, my motivation, I cannot carry out basic household stuff. It is very frustrating.'
>
> *Nancy*

Planning

Related to the unpredictability of symptoms is the uncertainty surrounding plans that you try to make. Such plans may have to be unmade. When symptoms are really bad, other people might have to take over duties at work and a partner might have to take over things for which you normally take responsibility. This can of course make people feel guilty, even to the extent that they stop making plans and become more reclusive, especially if they already have a fear of having symptoms when out socially (see Chapter 7 on how to overcome this fear of going out to public places). Uncertainty and unpredictability are highly disabling factors. You just want to be like everyone else, but everyone else looks fine!

But of course, we should remember that, out of all the people we meet, a good number of these will have either physical or psychological problems, which they hide well. They may indeed be suffering from IBS, but invisible chronic illness means we won't know. If you suffer from IBS you are not alone, even when you feel you are.

> 'I've had IBS for six years now (I'm 24) and it's such a lonely, debilitating illness. The biggest problem I have is not being able to get the symptoms under control (no tabs or diet have given me much relief) and my social life is basically non-existent as I'm always in discomfort and too depressed about finding places to eat out. I feel I just can't enjoy life when symptoms are out of control! My family and friends try to understand but they just don't know how bad it can be!'
>
> *Lucy*

Hiding your symptoms

> 'I don't tell anyone about my symptoms; they wouldn't understand, and I would feel embarrassed.'
>
> *Mary*

It is easy to understand why people with IBS (and other conditions) hide their symptoms. Most people like to blend in; they don't want to feel different. They don't want to draw attention to their disease, feeling that people might judge them as being lazy or a hypochondriac. Also, having to explain what IBS is like, perhaps multiple times, is very frustrating and it's worse if you feel you have to justify IBS when people have no understanding of it. People who don't know much about the condition might voice their opinion that it is simply the result of stress, or the wrong diet, or easily cured by eating particular foods, or that you just aren't coping very well. They might say all sorts of inappropriate things. Hiding symptoms often seems a lot easier. But hiding symptoms has its downsides too. The more people know about IBS and its effects on lives, the more information they have, the better for everyone with the condition. A lot of patients have felt better about themselves once they had come out about it. Only they can judge what's best for them.

Shame and embarrassment

Many research studies show that people with IBS, and other diseases focused around the gastrointestinal (GI) system, feel ashamed and embarrassed about their illness. Noises from the gut, possible smells, needing to go urgently to the toilet, are all things that people find embarrassing. Once you become an ill person, or a patient, the view you have of yourself changes. You may no longer trust your body and feel that it lets you down at inopportune moments.

You may feel different and blame yourself for what you did or did not do – even though you are not to blame for your illness any more than those who have cancer or a stroke are to blame for theirs. All sorts of factors right from childhood predispose people to certain illnesses; you are unlucky if you are one of those people. Any shame or embarrassment needs addressing, so that the person with IBS does not go on feeling these emotions. We give more information on how to deal with these feelings in Chapter 7 (page 107).

Perceived stigma

This is the negative emotion people feel when they have something about them that they perceive to be shameful or unacceptable. Some illnesses are more 'acceptable' than others. For instance, AIDS and mental illnesses are stigmatised more than cancer. Conditions where people have embarrassing symptoms also have stigma attached to them. In 2002 our team published an article about perceived stigma and quality of life in men and women with IBS[14]. We found that perceived stigma was associated with a reduced quality of life. This was also the case with inflammatory bowel disease at that time. Although we now know more about IBS than before, it seems that IBS and IBD still are associated with feelings of shame and stigma. In 2011, Tiffany Taft and colleagues carried out a study looking at over 400 people with IBS or IBD[15]. Their study was interesting, as they identified the *sources* of perceived stigma – that is, whether the stigma was felt to arise from friends, family, healthcare providers, spouses, co-workers or employers. Overall, those with IBS felt more stigmatised than those with IBD. They felt most stigmatised by friends, followed by healthcare providers, co-workers and employers, and least stigmatised by family and spouses. The study found that perceived stigma was associated with increased depression and anxiety.

'It does have a huge impact on my life as it is so unpredictable and I can go for ages feeling fine but it all of a sudden flares up again. I'm not a huge drinker but if my friends want to go out and I drink then I usually end the night with an awful stomach ache. I do tend to hide my symptoms, especially when they're embarrassing ones, such as gas, bloating and diarrhoea, which can happen all of a sudden. If I am at work and I get symptoms, I always try and find a toilet that is hidden or nowhere near any other people! It is really embarrassing, especially if people ask.'

Gemma

Relationships

Cecilia Håkanson and colleagues from Sweden have carried out studies on the various experiences that people with IBS have in relation to their disease. Their studies show clearly the ways they feel about their disease, and the ways in which it affects their lives and relationships.

Relationships with healthcare professionals

One study by this Swedish group looked at the experiences patients with IBS had of dealings with healthcare professionals[16]. Some had supportive encounters, but unfortunately more had unsupportive ones. In the unsupportive encounters, people were not taken seriously, healthcare professionals dismissed them or told them to 'calm down'. Sometimes they were told they were exaggerating or imagining their illness. Not being taken seriously is a recurring theme in the experiences of people with IBS. This is no doubt because the condition is *invisible*. In fact, the researchers said that they felt that looking ill would have been better, as then others would have taken them seriously. Their research found that they felt insignificant in their encounters with healthcare professionals, that they weren't believed, and that their feelings were not understood.

Supportive encounters included being acknowledged as a person – that is, the healthcare professional listened to the patient without judgement and developed a relationship based on respect and trust. The key to the development of trust was not to do with a doctor having extensive knowledge about IBS, but rather the practitioner's genuine interest in the patient's experience of symptoms and life with IBS. This shows that it is not necessary to see the top (and most probably most expensive!) professional in gastroenterology to have a good doctor–patient relationship and, in turn, appropriate medical care. Rather, the healthcare professional should be open and accepting of IBS and its effects on patients' lives. Hence, in this study supportive encounters with doctors led patients to feel that their feelings were legitimised.

Medical legitimisation

Medical legitimisation is a very important theme for us. The term refers to healthcare professionals and others believing you have a real illness which is important enough to consider seriously. Illnesses differ in the extent to which they have this legitimisation, and the invisible illnesses tend to be the ones which have low medical legitimisation, because if people can't see your illness, then they may doubt you are actually ill. Cancer probably has the highest medical legitimisation. Research shows that people who have an illness which isn't legitimised become more depressed and anxious than people whose illness is legitimised, even if they have similar symptoms.

> 'Until fairly recently, I was typically told it was a bout of diarrhoea that would pass, or that I had a bug of some sort. I didn't really connect all the dots myself, so I can't really blame medical professionals for being so slow on the uptake.'
>
> *Justin*

Relationships with friends and family

Medical legitimisation is one thing, but to have friends and family who validate and legitimise your illness is also important – maybe even more important. People with invisible illnesses are often more disappointed when their family and friends seem to doubt them, as when healthcare professionals doubt them. As attitudes towards IBS have become more positive, hopefully friends and family will be less likely to have negative attitudes.

Starting new intimate relationships

People with IBS are often worried about disclosing their problems to potential partners. They might fear rejection or be embarrassed to start talking about IBS – or perhaps not know how to broach the subject. There are many embarrassing illnesses, and, sadly, when bowel problems and toilets are involved, people are inevitably embarrassed. Really the best way of coping with this is to be honest about it from the beginning. Tell the potential partner how it affects you, but let him/her know that IBS is only one part of your life. Needless to say, if potential partners don't want to pursue a relationship just because you have IBS, then you've probably had a lucky escape. IBS is a medical disease just like other diseases and affects quality of life, even if it doesn't affect longevity.

Maintaining existing intimate relationships

'Finally I got the courage to tell my girlfriend I had IBS. She did know there was something wrong, but I told her that I was being investigated for colitis, which I thought sounded better. I was really worried about telling her, but she just said she knew a few people with IBS and so what? So then we were able to talk all about IBS and it was a real relief to know she understood. I wish I had told her earlier.'

Edward

Having a condition like IBS can wreak havoc with intimate relationships. Apart from feeling unattractive due to bloating, burbulence, wind and all the other symptoms that come with the condition, the fear of needing to use the loo during sexual encounters can kill a sex life. Constipation can also make sex painful for some women. Apart from using the treatment and self-help strategies to reduce symptoms that are described later in this book, communication about your fears can help you and your partner maintain intimacy and a sexual relationship. If your partner isn't supportive and understanding, it may be worth seeing a counsellor to help open the channels of communication. There is very little research about IBS and sexual relationships (and how to maintain them), but author and 'sexuality expert' Cory Silverberg has written a number of straightforward and practical articles, including issues surrounding bowel control during sex:

- http://sexuality.about.com/od/sex_and_disability/a/Bowel-And-Bladder-Control-During-Sex.htm – An introduction to how to approach bowel control during intimate contact

- http://sexuality.about.com/od/sex_and_disability/a/Tips-On-Talking-About-Bowel-And-Bladder-Control-During-Sex.htm – A guide to how to talk about bowel control during sex

- http://sexuality.about.com/od/tipstechniques/ht/Control-Bowel-And-Bladder-During-Sex.htm – How to deal with loss of bowel control during sex.

Reading these articles with or without your partner may help not just with sex *per se*, but all-round intimacy as some of Cory's ideas involve challenging our views of 'sexiness' and what sex really is – that is, not what is portrayed in the media but rather a quite messy and 'unsexy' thing altogether!

Why is social support important?

Social support has been found to have positive effects on the lives of people with IBS. You know how good it feels when people around you acknowledge your difficulties, when they accept you as you are and you know you can tell them anything and they will still support you. Social support from others is really important.

One recent study by Lackner and colleagues in the USA found that IBS patients who had high social support had less severe pain than those who had low social support[17]. In fact, people who had better support from others had less severe symptoms in general.

This is most likely due to a positive effect on the BGA/HPA system (page 13), as studies suggest that good social relationships can reduce the stress responses from this system. Social support can act as a protective factor against getting diseases (see Chapters 1 and 9 for more on the BGA/HPA system).

Why does social support have these beneficial effects? Well, it is partly hormonal. Oxytocin is a hormone which is secreted by the pituitary gland in the brain. It is involved in the regulation of childbirth and breast-feeding, strengthening the bond between mother and child. However, it has wider effects than this. Oxytocin is released when you feel supported by others. Studies have shown that oxytocin and social support interact together in reducing cortisol (a stress hormone), which means that stress is reduced. Heinrichs and colleagues at the University of Trier in Germany carried out a study in which men with and without social support were either injected with oxytocin or a placebo[18]. All were first subjected to a stressful task – in this case, public speaking and solving mental arithmetic problems in front of an audience. The researchers then measured the levels of cortisol in the men and collected information on how anxious or calm they felt via questionnaires. The researchers found that men with no social support had high levels of cortisol and also had a decrease in calmness and increase in anxiety levels. Those who had social support or oxytocin (or both) were calmer after the stressful experience and had less anxiety.

Working life

Employers now have to make reasonable adjustments for people with medical conditions. So, for instance, a person with a bad back might need a special chair; someone with ME/CFS might need to have more rest breaks. If your IBS is worse in the morning, your employer might agree for you to start work later. You are the best person to determine your needs, so you need to tell your employer that you have IBS and how it affects you, so that managers can make any adjustments to your working practices. This might mean having an office near the toilets, or needing flexibility in terms of sick leave, working hours or work breaks.

Employers are not allowed to discriminate against you because of any medical conditions, and many employers are extremely helpful and supportive of people with long-term medical conditions. Obviously you can ask your employer to keep your medical problems confidential.

Is IBS classified as a disability?

Under the Equality Act 2010 a person is classified as disabled if they have a physical or mental impairment which has a substantial and long-term effect on their ability to carry out normal day-to-day activities.

If you cannot work

If the IBS is severe and restricts a person so much that he/she can't work, then it could be considered a disability. If it has a substantial and long-term negative effect, such that a person can't work, it might be possible to apply for a benefit called the Personal Independence Payment (PIP). It will involve an assessment where certain conditions have to be met:

- be aged 16 to 64
- have a long-term health condition (more than 12 months) or disability and difficulties with activities related to daily living and/or mobility
- be in Great Britain when you claim – there are some exceptions, e.g. members of the Armed Forces and their family members
- have been in Great Britain for at least two of the last three years
- be habitually resident in the UK, Ireland, Isle of Man or the Channel Islands
- not be subject to immigration control (unless you're a sponsored immigrant)

For further information, see https://www.gov.uk/pip/eligibility.

Depression and stress

> 'My doctor told me that stress is a big factor for anyone with IBS but I really don't remember having any stressful times … I was a stay-at-home mum (thank god). To be honest, the thought of going out away from my home (and toilet) was causing the MOST stress … people who don't suffer from IBS don't understand that … it's not stress, it's FEAR.'
>
> *Danielle*

Some people might be told, or feel, that they are depressed. People with IBS, and others who have invisible chronic diseases, do show a higher rate of depression than people who are healthy. This seems likely to be true, since living with a chronic illness, which is often misunderstood and which seems to have no particular cause or cure, *is* depressing. It's very hard to be constantly happy and optimistic when you are ill. People with a cold or flu are likely to feel dreadful too, even though they know the virus will be gone in a short time. It's much worse if you don't know how long your symptoms will last.

If you or someone you know feels depressed rather than simply low, it is best to deal with the depression by going to the GP and perhaps accepting antidepressants. Some antidepressants calm the bowel and can help you sleep. Do discuss this with your doctor, however, as certain antidepressants can also irritate your stomach.

Fatigue and sleep

> 'Living with the symptoms every single day leads to stress and fatigue. I don't sleep well now, and I worry a lot, which makes the pain worse I think. I used to just take medications but now I've bought some CDs for relaxation and those have helped me.'
>
> *Nicola*

The problems that people with IBS have are similar to those of people with other invisible conditions. IBS, ME/CFS, Meniere's disease, fibromyalgia etc all have some symptoms in common. The main ones are fatigue and sleep problems. Fatigue is a key symptom of ME/CFS, but is a factor in most illnesses.

Fatigue can be a result of the following:

- side effects of medications given to help the symptoms

- sleep deprivation: having an illness sometimes leads to poor sleep due to symptoms and illness-related worries

- cytokines being produced in your body as a result of your illness, the side effects of which include tiredness

- trying to ignore the symptoms so that you can meet all your commitments and responsibilities, instead of ensuring you have enough rest and relaxation.

These factors, and having such intrusive physical symptoms, means you might not be getting enough good quality sleep. This might be because the symptoms themselves wake you up, or that you wake up and begin to worry, perhaps because you fear you might lose your job, or that you won't be able to cope, or that you might have a different disease to that of IBS. Sleep is really important for healthy people, and for people with chronic illness, it is especially important.

The actual length of time you sleep predicts how healthy you are – and lack of sleep (less than five hours) has been shown to lead to health problems such as obesity, stroke, diabetes, anxiety and depression. Job stress has been shown to affect quality of sleep; in a study of nurses, for example, the higher the level of job strain, the less they slept.

In terms of IBS, studies show that people report decreased sleep duration and quality and that they feel fatigued during the day. IBS symptoms are worse when sleep quality or quantity are worse. One study in particular found that after a bad night's sleep symptoms of IBS were worse the next morning[19]. People who have high levels of social support have a better quality of sleep than those with less support. Conversely, people who find that their friends are not supportive and that these friends only created stress for them, were more likely to suffer from disturbed sleep.

> 'I have problems sleeping. It used to be just staying asleep was an issue as I had no problems falling asleep, but now I have problems getting to sleep as well … I did finally get a prescription for sleeping pills from my doctor but they only let me get maybe four straight hours. I have not had a good night's sleep (without meds) in probably 10 years or more.'
>
> *Danielle*

Lack of sleep affects the immune system and can activate an inflammatory response. Not getting enough sleep can also mean that your immune system is less able to mount a response to a viral infection, so if you sleep badly you might be more prone to coughs and colds.

People who have never experienced true fatigue might be sympathetic but they cannot really put themselves in your position. Fatigue can affect both work life and home life. Work life is, of necessity, the first thing to protect, so a person may go flat out to make sure no one realises how bad they feel. When something has to give, it's home life, hobbies, and social outings. Relationships with partners and family can often be strained, especially if a partner has to take on additional responsibilities when you are too ill to do them.

The stress and worry of coping with a chronic illness has biological and physiological effects, not just psychological (see Chapter 1). We give advice on how to deal with anxiety and stress in Chapter 7. We also give tips on how to get a better night's sleep in Chapter 4.

Summary

In this chapter we've discussed IBS as a condition that has a substantial and long-term effect on both personal and working life. We have suggested that people should tell their employers so that they can give support in work and that if a person wants to work but cannot as IBS symptoms are too bad, then it is possible to apply for state benefits (if you are in the UK). We have discussed the ways in which IBS can affect different aspects of a person's life, including relationships with healthcare professionals, friends and family. As IBS is an invisible illness it can be hard for people to understand how terrible someone with the condition feels, the embarrassment associated with gastrointestinal symptoms and the fear that goes with possibly having an accident in public. In the next chapter we are going to look at some of the tests and procedures that a doctor might request in order to diagnose IBS and also things that can be done to help a doctor reach an accurate diagnosis.

Chapter 3

Diagnosis of IBS: what to expect

'Before I was diagnosed I was experiencing the effects of IBS almost daily, and it was causing me a lot of anxiety. I didn't know much about IBS and was really worried that the symptoms I was experiencing might be the signs of something really serious. I was too scared to search online for answers as I was worried what it might say. It came as quite a relief to me when I was told what I had could be managed and was given advice about treatments I could use that would help.'

Kwilole

When you have IBS, it can feel that you're completely at sea, awash in symptoms, mistrusting your own body and not knowing where to turn for help. The first step in finding the right treatment package is gaining a diagnosis. In this chapter we outline some of the tests a doctor might request in order to diagnose your symptoms. We also look at ways to help the doctor diagnose what's going on, such as completing a symptom diary. Even people already diagnosed with IBS may find the material in this chapter useful as we also talk about procedures that may happen if they ever see a specialist gastroenterologist. Don't worry, however, if you think you have IBS but haven't had all of these procedures as you'll only be asked to undergo them if your doctor thinks there's good reason to – for example, to rule out other conditions that may explain the symptoms.

GP consultation

'After a bad flare-up and years of struggling with symptoms I again went to see the doctor, a new doctor this time. I was at the end of my tether by this point. A junior doctor, he was very 'thorough'. He asked me a long list of questions, examined my abdomen and conducted a series of blood tests and eventually concluded that I had IBS.'

Justin

The GP will see many people in her surgery who say they have gastrointestinal symptoms. To decide whether their symptoms are due to IBS or something else, she will ask for a history of the problem, which may include a number of questions along these lines:

- Have you had abdominal pain or bloating that seems to go away when you have a bowel movement?

- Does your abdominal pain or bloating seem to happen at the same time as periods of diarrhoea or constipation?

- Have you been passing more stools than you usually do?

The GP will also ask for a time frame for these symptoms, such as have they just started or have they been going on for some months? Some other questions that the GP may ask are:

- Have you needed to strain when you pass stools, when you didn't previously?

- Have you been experiencing a sense of urgency or feeling you have not emptied your bowels properly that is new for you when going to the toilet?

- Do you have any hardness or tension in your abdomen?

- Are your symptoms worse after eating?

- Have you noticed any mucus from your back passage when you go to the toilet?

Many GPs will diagnose IBS based on the answers to these types of question and whether the symptoms fit into the 'Rome criteria' as mentioned in Chapter 1 (page 11). If you have only recently had these symptoms, sometimes the GP will tell you she suspects that you have IBS, but to monitor your symptoms (often with a symptom diary – see below in this chapter, page 48) to determine whether certain activities or foods aggravate your symptoms. She may offer you medication for diarrhoea or constipation, or an antidepressant. These are sometimes given as they have an analgesic (pain relieving) effect and also help with sleep. She may therefore give a prescription for antidepressants whether or not she thinks you are depressed.

If you are young and reasonably fit (apart from your IBS symptoms), the GP may ask you to come back in a few weeks if symptoms haven't resolved. In order to be diagnosed with IBS, you need to have had the symptoms for around six months.

If you have been asked to monitor your symptoms and come back in a few weeks, then the best thing to do is to keep a symptom diary and to try to discover when your symptoms are worse and when they get better. Also, if you have been prescribed any medications, to take them as directed and note down whether or not they help your symptoms.

Your GP may ask you for a stool sample, a blood test and a breath test. She may also do a rectal examination to check for haemorrhoids ('piles').

Stool test

The stool sample will be checked for colour, consistency, amount, shape, odour and the presence of mucus. It may also be examined for parasites, hidden blood, fat, meat fibres, bile, white blood cells and sugars, which may help your doctor figure out why you've been having GI symptoms. The stool test can also help to rule out inflammatory bowel disease (see Chapter 1, page 7). A 'stool culture' may be performed too in order to look for bacteria.

Full blood count

A full blood count (FBC) looks at the following components of the blood:

- *Erythrocyte sedimentation rate (ESR)*: This test will show whether you have any inflammation anywhere in the body. It can't tell the GP where the inflammation is, but it's just one piece of information that can be useful, along with other results, such as the 'CRP' below.

- *C-reactive protein (CRP)*: This is a substance produced in the liver. It also shows whether or not there is inflammation in the body.

- *White blood cell count*: This can show whether you have an infection.

- *Red blood cell count*: This shows whether you have anaemia of one sort or another.

Rectal examination

Most people will find a rectal (back passage) examination embarrassing but your doctor or nurse will be aware of this. If for whatever reason (religious, cultural or simply personal preference) you would like the examination performed by someone who is the same sex as you, let the receptionist know before the day of your appointment for this. If you've not been given prior notice of this exam but would like a same-sex doctor or nurse to perform it, it is fine to ask for another appointment with an alternative practitioner. During the examination you will need to remove your clothing from the waist down and lie on your side on a medical table or couch with your knees pulled upwards to your chest. The doctor will first look for obvious abnormalities, like warts, rashes, haemorrhoids ('piles' – swollen blood vessels around the anus or rectum that can cause bleeding) or any skin tears near your back passage. Next the doctor will gently push a finger into your bottom and then further up your rectum. This can be uncomfortable and may cause some pain but the doctor will use lubrication (and gloves for hygiene) to make the procedure easier for you. The doctor might ask you to squeeze the muscles in your rectum so that she/he can see if they're working properly. If you're a man, the doctor might also perform a prostate examination at this time, which involves pressing on the prostate gland. This shouldn't hurt but it may make you want to pass urine or feel a little tender. This entire procedure shouldn't take more than five minutes and often considerably less, so while it's not pleasant, it should be quick.

Antibody test for coeliac disease

People who have coeliac disease (sensitivity to wheat and other gluten-containing grains) have symptoms that resemble IBS (see Chapter 1, page 7). A blood test would let your GP know whether or not you have coeliac disease.

Breath tests

A breath test can tell whether you have **bacterial overgrowth** (see Chapter 9, page 137).

It can also show whether you are intolerant to lactose as this results in similar symptoms to those of IBS if you eat or drink anything with lactose in it. Lactose is a sugar found in dairy products, such as cow's milk, butter, and cheese, and people who are lactose intolerant do not have enough of an important enzyme called lactase. If you have this problem, then a lactose-free diet will help you, and you may no longer be diagnosed as having IBS.

Diagnosis of food allergies

Skin-prick testing or blood test

A skin-prick test is a quick test to determine whether you are allergic to food allergens. The skin will be punctured on your arm, and a tiny bit of allergen will be introduced. If you are allergic, then a red spot will appear within a few minutes as a result of the release of 'histamine', a substance that is an important part of the immune response.

Sometimes a blood test will be taken and later analysed to see whether you have a reaction to the production of 'immunoglobulin E' (IgE) antibodies in reaction to certain foods. If you do have a reaction, then you will know you are allergic to these foods and can take steps to manage this problem (see Chapter 5, page 72).

Food challenges

Under close supervision, you will be given a small amount of the foods to which you suspect you are allergic, in order to see what happens. If you are allergic to the food, then you can be given treatment straight away to counter your allergic response. We discuss food allergies in more detail in Chapter 5.

Food intolerance and sensitivities

There are no mainstream diagnostic tests (i.e. tests that you can get from your GP) which can show you whether or not you are intolerant or sensitive to certain foods. However, a number of private clinics offer specialised testing which claims to identify trigger foods so you may want to consider visiting one such clinic. Please do bear in mind this form of testing can be quite expensive and there is not a great deal of independent research to support its use, although this may of course change in time once more research is carried out. However, you can use an exclusion, or elimination, diet to discover if you are sensitive or intolerant to particular foods and drinks. In Chapter 5 there is guidance on how to do this.

Further testing

If a member of your family has had certain types of cancer (bowel or ovarian), your GP may also want to run more tests on you. If you are middle-aged or older, it is also more likely you will be offered further tests to determine whether you have IBS or something more serious. This is because the likelihood of other illnesses, such as inflammatory bowel disease or bowel cancer, is higher in older people.

Whatever your age, you may have some 'red flag' symptoms that will prompt your GP to carry out more tests. These include:

- Weight loss that cannot be explained by any other cause, such as a change in diet or lifestyle

- Obvious swelling or a lump in your abdomen or back passage (rectum)

- Bleeding from your back passage (rectum)

- Anaemia (low red blood cell count).

If your GP decides you should have further tests, she will refer you to a gastroenterologist.

Procedures

If you've been referred to a specialist there are a number of procedures that you may be asked to undertake. There's no point trying to hide the fact that these can be unpleasant. No one wants to experience intrusive medical procedures in intimate areas, but these will generally be uncomfortable at most, not painful, and the results will help your gastroenterologist decide the best course of action for your treatment, which can only be a positive thing in the long run.

Sigmoidoscopy

One of the first tests you might be offered is a sigmoidoscopy, which is a procedure that is carried out in the hospital or the GP's surgery. It doesn't require an overnight stay and you can usually go home soon after the test. This procedure involves a sigmoidoscope, which is a thin, flexible tube that has a small camera and light attached.

This is inserted into the rectum so that the gastroenterologist can investigate your lower bowel. This is to see if there are any polyps or signs of cancerous growths. Bowel polyps are small growths (usually less than 1 cm) that are not normally cancerous but may need to be removed to make sure they don't turn into cancer. Polyps are very common – it is thought about 15-20% of people in the UK have them – and most people don't notice them at all as they often don't cause symptoms.

People don't normally need sedatives for a sigmoidoscopy and the actual test only takes between 10-20 minutes. It might be uncomfortable (as you can imagine), but it shouldn't be painful. The gastroenterologist will start by examining your rectum (see page 38). You'll be asked to lie on your left side with your knees bent to make this easier. Once the sigmoidoscope has been gently inserted, carbon dioxide gas or air is pumped into the lower bowel which makes it expand. This makes it easier for the gastroenterologist to view the bowel wall with the instrument but may be a bit uncomfortable as you may feel like you need to pass wind or go to the toilet; this is completely normal and you shouldn't feel embarrassed.

Your gastroenterologist will at this stage be looking at a video monitor where the pictures of your bowel are displayed. If she sees polyps she may want to remove them there and then and this shouldn't cause you any pain. She may also want to take a biopsy which will be looked at later in the hospital laboratory.

It is best to rest at home after a sigmoidoscopy, but there is very little chance of significant side effects from this procedure. You may feel bloated for a few hours or have stomach cramps, but these should pass. If they do not, please tell your GP. If you've had polyps removed or if the gastroenterologist took a biopsy, you may experience some bleeding from the rectum. This should stop within a few days, but if the bleeding becomes heavy, please contact your GP and the hospital where the test was carried out.

Barium enema

If the sigmoidoscopy or routine blood tests are abnormal, you may be offered a barium enema. This procedure is unlikely to be painful, but it can be uncomfortable.

Before you have this procedure, you will be given a leaflet telling you what you should or should not eat, in order to ensure that your bowel is emptied; and to make extra sure this happens, you will also be asked to take laxatives.

You will be seen in the X-ray department of the hospital. Normally a needle will be inserted in your arm in order to be given mild sedation.

A milky substance (barium – a substance that shows up when X-rayed) is pumped up through your rectum and through to your colon. This contains air as well as the barium. Your bowel, and the passage of the barium through the bowel, can be seen as X-rays on a computer monitor.

The radiographer will later look at the images in detail, to determine whether anything unusual, like tumours or inflammation, is present. This means waiting a few days for the results.

If you have IBS, everything should show up as normal – which doesn't mean 'there's nothing wrong with you'. There is something wrong, but at this point the diagnosis may still be uncertain.

Upper GI series

A barium swallow and meal involves swallowing a drink that contains barium (a substance which shows up on X-rays). The barium coats the inside of your throat, oesophagus (the pipe that goes from your mouth to your stomach), stomach and small bowel. This allows for clearer X-ray images.

You will have to refrain from eating for a few hours before the test. The doctors might tell you the barium drink is like a milk shake, and it does look like that, but unfortunately it doesn't taste like one. Once you have drunk the chalk-like drink, after a short pause, the radiographer will take X-rays of the upper part of your gastrointestinal (GI) system. The barium meal moves down through your throat, oesophagus, stomach and small bowel; and the images are recorded. Later the radiographer will look at the images in detail in order to determine whether any tumours or ulcers are present in the upper part of the GI system.

Upper endoscopy

This is a procedure where an 'endoscope' will be used in order to look at the lining of your upper GI tract. The endoscope is a long flexible tube with a tiny camera attached. An anaesthetic will ensure that your throat is numb; the endoscope will be passed down your oesophagus and into your stomach and duodenum (the first section of your small bowel). You can choose to be sedated for this procedure. The doctor will be able to see any abnormalities in the upper GI tract.

Colonoscopy

'For me the preparation for the colonoscopy was the worst part. This was because before the procedure I had to take some strong laxatives (which were provided by the hospital). This meant that I couldn't go very far from a toilet for two days. There's no avoiding this because your bowels have to be totally empty before the test. If you're on any medication then your doctor may advise you to stop taking these before the procedure. I had to stop taking iron supplements because they make the inside of the bowel go black which would have meant the doctor would not have been able to see anything. I was told in advance that many patients have no memory of the colonoscopy procedure due to the sedative given.

'The actual procedure wasn't too bad. I had mine done as a day patient. I was given some trousers with a hole at the back to wear, and I was given some painkillers and a sedative. It started with me lying on my side and then at different points the doctor turned me over from side to side, but the sedative worked so well that I was only vaguely aware of what was happening. It's difficult to really remember what it was like to have the colonoscopy. I remember the intravenous injection and then nothing much apart from seeing lots of bright colours swirling around like a kaleidoscope and the next thing that I knew was I was in the recovery room. The same thing happened when I had the endoscopy. Afterwards I was given time for the sedation to wear off and then went home (escorted – hospitals won't let patients out alone after they've had sedation).'

Liz

Sometimes, especially if people are middle-aged or older, the GP will refer them to the clinic or hospital to have a colonoscopy, rather than having a barium enema and sigmoidoscopy. A colonoscopy is similar to a sigmoidoscopy, but in this procedure a device called a colonoscope is used. This instrument is longer than a sigmoidoscope and so can see inside the length of your bowel (large intestine) This enables the gastroenterologist to determine whether polyps or cancer are present anywhere in the length of the bowel. This test takes around 30–35 minutes to complete and you will be offered a sedative or painkiller to make sure you're as comfortable as possible during the procedure. You will be asked to lie on your left-hand side so that the doctor can insert the colonoscope, or 'endoscope', into your back passage (rectum), with the aid of lubricant.

As with the sigmoidoscopy, some air will be pumped inside your bowel so that the colonoscope can pass through the bowel with ease, which might cause wind. This will feel strange but try not to worry about it; it is simply part of the procedure. Also like the sigmoidoscopy the doctor will view your bowel on a monitor and possibly take a biopsy or remove polyps. You won't feel any pain however and you may not actually remember much about the procedure due to the effects of the sedative, as per Liz's account above.

Aftercare is the same as for the sigmoidoscopy so keep an eye out for any excess bleeding or discomfort. But if you have had a sedative you will need to rest immediately afterwards to allow it to wear off; also, arrange for someone to collect you from the hospital. Don't drive, drink alcohol, operate heavy machinery or make any important decisions for at least 24 hours after the procedure as sedative can impair your judgement and cognitive abilities. After 24 hours you should be back to normal and able to return to your daily activities.

Ultrasound

An ultrasound scanner is able to provide moving pictures of particular organs. You might have an abdominal scan and/or a pelvic scan. For the scans, you will be lying down. The sonographer (who performs the ultrasound) will put a gel over your abdomen and/or pelvis. She then moves a sensor around the appropriate areas, which produces pictures which she can see on a computer screen. You might also be able to look at the screen.

The actual procedure differs according to the type of scan. For some, you might have to drink water beforehand, so that your bladder is full when you have the scan. This is not a problem unless there is some delay at the hospital, and you have to wait a lot longer than expected – then you might have to go to the loo! If this happens, and you cannot stop mid-stream, then the appointment might need to be rescheduled.

For other types of scan, you might have to not eat anything for some while beforehand, or you might have to keep your bladder empty. You will be given all the appropriate instructions in advance of the appointment. None of these procedures is unpleasant or painful, and you will be able to go straight home afterwards.

Although the scan can't diagnose IBS, it will be able to rule out other problems, such as gall stones, cysts and abscesses.

Working with your doctor

So far in this chapter we have looked in detail at the questions you are likely to be asked by your GP, the tests that you may have in primary care and the likely procedures you will undergo if you're referred to a specialist. This may seem overwhelming or, on the other hand, you may feel frustrated if your doctor has not referred you for more tests.

With a complex illness like IBS that may take time to diagnose, it's important to try to develop a collaborative relationship with your GP. This is, of course, a two-way process and if you feel your GP isn't taking your concerns and symptoms seriously, ask if any other doctor in the practice has a special interest in gastrointestinal disorders as s/he will have more up-to-date knowledge of IBS. (In Chapter 8 we will look at medical professionals' views of IBS and how these can differ from patients' ideas about their symptoms.)

There are a few ways to develop a collaborative relationship with the doctor which help her to make an accurate diagnosis:

- Keep a detailed symptom diary (below)

- Don't expect a diagnosis straight away – IBS is diagnosed on the basis of symptoms and the exclusion of other diseases so this may take time; try to be patient even though this may be hard

- Be active in taking control of your condition – IBS is a complex disorder and as such you may need to use a combination of symptom-relief medications, stress-reduction techniques and other changes to your daily patterns and habits (which we will discuss in Chapters 4–7). This does not mean that you are to blame in any way at all for having IBS, rather that there are many things that you can do yourself to manage your symptoms.

Tracking symptoms with an IBS diary

'Keep a regular journal of your triggers – whether it's certain foods, a particular time of the month or nerve-wracking situations, it will all be useful in helping you manage the condition on an ongoing basis. Keeping a diary will make it really clear when and why IBS affects you personally.'

Nicola

In order to help identify trigger foods and daily stresses that may exacerbate your IBS, it is extremely useful to keep records of symptoms and activities in a personal IBS diary. A symptom diary for IBS differs from versions for other conditions as you need to pay particular attention to the nature and types of IBS symptoms you have and also to exactly what you're eating. Many of us are quite unaware of what we eat and can be rather surprised when we look at it on paper. Also, trying to simply recall foods, drinks, symptoms and everyday stresses is not at all easy. Therefore, a detailed diary can help both you and your doctor identify any patterns in your IBS that will help healthcare professionals come up with an effective treatment plan.

Bristol stool chart

Before we outline what an IBS diary should look like, you need to know how to identify your bowel movement type. This might sound unpleasant and embarrassing, but the characteristics of your bowel movements can provide important information about your gastrointestinal health, especially if your stools change over time.

The Bristol stool chart (Figure 2), based on the Bristol Stool Form Scale, was developed at the University Department of Medicine in Bristol's Royal Infirmary by Dr Kenneth Heaton (now sadly deceased but he played a major part in helping scientists and doctors understand and be able to diagnose IBS). The chart contains seven different stool types that vary in size and shape, from small hard lumps (think rabbit poos) to completely liquid diarrhoea (see below).

Types 1 and 2 are indicative of constipation and difficult to pass. Types 3 and 4 show more healthy bowel movements and shouldn't require straining (but it's important to bear in mind that everyone is different and you can have any combination of sensations and stool type – what matters is what's normal for you and if this suddenly changes). Types 5–7 are often accompanied by the urgent need to go to the toilet and suggest mild to severe diarrhoea. You can use these classifications in your IBS diary to help your doctor understand your individual bowel habits.

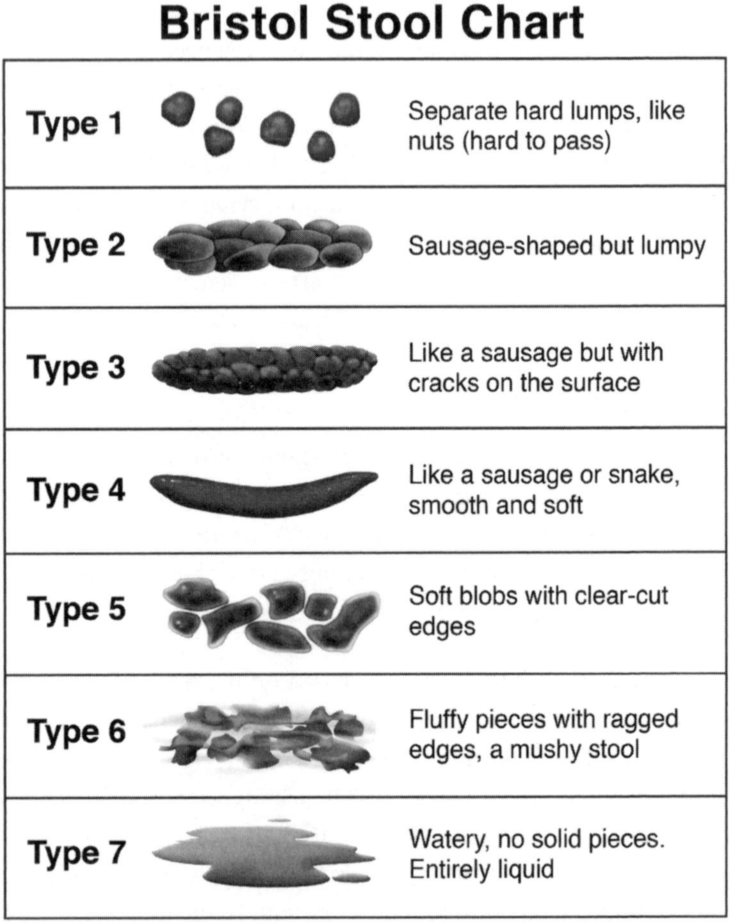

Bristol Stool Chart

Type 1		Separate hard lumps, like nuts (hard to pass)
Type 2		Sausage-shaped but lumpy
Type 3		Like a sausage but with cracks on the surface
Type 4		Like a sausage or snake, smooth and soft
Type 5		Soft blobs with clear-cut edges
Type 6		Fluffy pieces with ragged edges, a mushy stool
Type 7		Watery, no solid pieces. Entirely liquid

Figure 2 The Bristol Stool Chart – This is a useful tool in helping to identify types of bowel movements; this information can help doctors to diagnose IBS-like symptoms. (Copyright © 2006. Rome Foundation. All rights reserved.)

IBS symptom and food diary

There are numerous versions of IBS symptom diaries online, apps that can be downloaded on smartphones and tablets and paper-based methods that can be purchased, but of course you can simply use a paper and pen to construct a diary. The key areas to include are:

- Today's date and day of the week – it doesn't matter which day it starts on but including this somewhat obvious piece of information helps in case any of the pages get muddled up. Also, symptoms could follow a weekly pattern if there are any triggers that occur on specific days; for instance a coffee morning with friends or tense weekly meetings at work (even if you are unable to do these things do keep a record of the date as very small daily changes may be affecting the IBS).

- You can use a grid where rows are time points and columns are categories to note, as below in Figure 3, or simply use a different sheet of paper for each of the events.

To summarise the table on page 52, the categories you need to include in your IBS diary, or check are in the app or downloaded version that you want to use, are:

- bowel movement type (see stool chart above), whether you felt you hadn't been able to pass all the faeces (known as an 'incomplete evacuation') or incontinence (having an accident)

- pain – for example, pain on either side of your abdomen, stomach cramping, lower intestinal cramping, tenderness (when the skin is pressed), rectal pain (note down whether this pain is sharp, dull, burning), other rectal pain such as the sensation of a hard object in the rectum or cramping in the rectum

- other GI symptoms – for example, burbulence, belching, passing wind; also describe any smell associated with the latter

- medication use – try to record the dose taken and the strength of tablets. Also include any herbal remedies, probiotics or prebiotics

- food and drink – it's important here to be as detailed as possible and include *everything* you eat and drink. The doctor is not going to judge your diet in terms of healthy/unhealthy, just

Event time	Bowel movement type	Pain	Other symptoms	Medication use	Food / drink	Feelings and stressors
wake time: 6.13		Sharp pain on left hand side, below tummy				Feeling really tired, not refreshed at all
6.14			Wind – strong egg-like smell			
6.15		Stomach cramps		Paracetamol 2 x 500mg		
6.22						Feeling anxious as woke up with symptoms and I need to get the kids to school – worried
6.23					Large cup of coffee with milk and 2 sugars	about symptoms on the way. Worried about eating anything before school run
6.25				Buscopan 2 x 10mg		
6.33	Strong urge to go then Type 6					
6.37			Uncomfortable belching immediately after BM			Dreading the day ahead
9.32					Crumpets x 2 with butter	Started to feel starving after BM so ate something plain after school run
Sleep time: 23.31						Feeling worried about marriage as feel too unattractive for sex (bloated tummy)

Figure 3 Symptom and food diary – This diary can be used by both patients and doctors to identify any patterns or triggers that might be associated with IBS symptoms

whether certain foods and beverages may be impacting on your IBS. The time and pattern are also important – for instance, in the example symptom diary above, our hypothetical person drank coffee on an empty stomach soon after waking. The reason for this is clear – she needed some 'get up and go' but was scared to eat anything before taking her children to school so had a caffeinated drink instead. The type of drink and also the delay in eating breakfast might be making her IBS symptoms worse, so noting down not just what food or drink but when and also why allows a healthcare professional to start to build a picture of your particular eating style and if there are any trigger foods/drinks

- feelings and stressors – write down how you're feeling when you wake up and go to bed as this may indicate a sleep problem that you may want to discuss with your doctor. Also, include any feelings associated with your IBS (or not), such as frustration, fear of eating, drinking, travelling etc. Other things to include in this column are stressors, such as a difficult presentation at work, arguments, daily obligations (work, shopping, childcare, cooking, etc), and more significant issues such as physical injuries, caring responsibilities, relationship or money worries, moving house or bereavement.

You may also want to add an additional column or page to report exercise, symptoms of any other illnesses or infection and medications for these (for instance antibiotics can cause stomach upset), cigarettes or other smoking products, if you smoke, and your menstrual cycle if you're a woman. Aim to complete your IBS diary for two to four weeks so that there is enough time to see patterns emerge.

As you can see, an IBS diary will hold a great deal of information and may feel time-consuming and intrusive. However, the more accurate you can be, the more clues you and your doctor will have to the underlying nature of your IBS. This can take out some of the guess work and experimentation with different treatments; hence you'll be able to control your symptoms and get back to your life more quickly and also manage any subsequent flare-ups you may have in the future more effectively.

'I've been struggling with IBS symptoms for years now. But it's only recently, following diagnosis in November 2014, that I've started thinking about the problems I've had over the years as being related to IBS. Before that I wasn't sure what I had. In fact, I probably thought constant bloating, stomach cramps, mucousy diarrhoea and the various other bowel-based treats that go hand-in-hand with IBS were somehow "normal". Like everybody suffered the same problems all the time like I did.'

Justin

Summary

This chapter has included a lot of detail about what the doctor might ask in a consultation and some of the tests that might be performed either by a GP or a specialist. We have also outlined ways of gathering information to help doctors and other healthcare professionals to diagnose and then treat IBS (or other conditions if, after the consultations and tests, you are diagnosed with something else). This can seem overwhelming but it isn't necessary to take it in all at once – diagnosis is a process and everyone will have their own personal journey.

The next chapter is the first of four that outline treatments and other strategies to help deal with the symptoms of IBS.

Chapter 4

Medical treatments and other recommendations

'Making a positive diagnosis of IBS has several important implications: to reassure the patient; to make him or her feel confident about future decisions; to direct treatment and use resources in a logical manner.'

Mearin and Lacy[20]

It may at first seem strange that two people with IBS will be prescribed different medicines and given different advice about managing their illness. However, even though two people may have the same diagnosis, they could have had different triggers for IBS and there may also be different mechanisms leading to IBS symptoms in different people (this will be explored in Chapter 9). Even within one person, symptoms can vary from day to day, week to week or seem to change with the seasons. Therefore, you may need to try a number of options to find the best route for you. In addition, since at present there is no 'cure' for IBS, medical practitioners often advise targeting the symptoms separately. You may need to be patient when searching for effective treatments and once again it would be beneficial to complete an IBS diary so that any improvements or deterioration following treatments can be recorded. But don't lose hope – it *is* possible to find a combination of medicines and treatments that will allow you to start living a full life again.

Medications

Before we start to outline the medicines used to treat IBS symptoms, it's important to appreciate that these are not 'magic pills' – they are not cures in themselves (we wish it were that straightforward). Nevertheless, medications can be used in conjunction with other strategies (covered in Chapters 5, 6 and 7) to restore daily life. The effectiveness of these medications may depend on whether you have IBS-D, IBS-C, or an alternating pattern of diarrhoea and constipation. Most drugs have side effects and might interact with other medications you are taking. For instance, a lot of the medications discussed below have sedative effects. That means that taking alcohol with these drugs could increase the sedative effect. Driving or operating machinery could therefore be dangerous in such cases. Your doctor or pharmacist should tell you about any possible side effects of prescribed and over-the-counter medicines and each medication will list potential side effects in its information sheet. If you're unclear or concerned about side effects of medicines, discuss this with your doctor or pharmacist.

Some medications have been found to be effective for people who have diarrhoea, constipation and/or an alternation of the two. These are: tricyclic antidepressants, selective serotonin reuptake inhibitors, and antispasmodic medications.

Tricyclic antidepressants (TCAs)

People sometimes think, when their GP suggests trying anti-depressants, that the GP believes they are depressed. However, these medications can improve all the symptoms of IBS, whether the patient is depressed or not. A typical tricyclic antidepressant is amitriptyline, which calms the bowel and improves abdominal pain (you can also use over-the-counter pain relievers – discuss with your doctor or pharmacist if you are taking other medications, and always follow the dosage advice). In fact, this drug can be used to treat intense pain and therefore is often prescribed for people with chronic conditions such as ME/CFS or fibromyalgia. This medication may be prescribed in one dose at night, which helps sleep. If you are prescribed it for use during the day, note that these drugs have the sedative effect I mentioned before, so you will need to get used to their effects on your body before driving or operating machinery. Most drugs have side effects that affect some people and not others. The most common side effect from taking a TCA is a dry mouth, but you will find others listed in the patient leaflet that comes with the drug.

Selective serotonin reuptake inhibitors (SSRIs)

SSRIs are a newer form of antidepressant than tricyclic antidepressants and have fewer side effects. Like TCAs, they may be prescribed for people with IBS regardless of whether the patient is depressed. As their name suggests, they block the reuptake of a substance called serotonin in the brain; serotonin is a neurotransmitter associated with positive mood and relaxation.

Antispasmodic medications

These drugs reduce the spasms in your gut, so are often used to help IBS. Although peppermint oil isn't a drug, it also seems to help people with different types of IBS. It can improve abdominal pain, incomplete evacuation, urgency to have a bowel movement and bloating.

There are other drugs that also help reduce gut spasms and improve

IBS. Buscopan is a common one and is often prescribed for people with IBS and can also be purchased without a prescription at chemists in the UK. (In some countries this medication is prescription only.) Buscopan is now marketed as *IBS Relief* but it does not tackle all the symptoms of IBS, just the abdominal cramps, pain and discomfort, so you will need other strategies or medications to deal with constipation and diarrhoea.

> '*Buscopan IBS Relief* has been a breakthrough. Discovering that it can take away the one thing that I felt I had no control over and just had to bear, was brilliant!'
>
> *Emily*

Another type of antispasmodic medication often prescribed for IBS is Mebeverine. Antispasmodic medicines have similar side effects to TCAs. Again you should allow time to get used to the effects of these medications before you drive or operate machinery.

Medications for specific symptoms

Diarrhoea

Loperamide is a fast-acting drug which slows down activity in the bowel and is thus useful for IBS-D. It has also been found to improve abdominal pain and overall symptoms. In the UK this is an over-the-counter drug, and most individuals with IBS do not report any adverse side effects. However, if you take too much of this medication you might then find you have constipation.

Bulk-forming agents, such as Ispaghula (see below), are also helpful for diarrhoea.

Constipation

With all treatments for constipation you should drink plenty of water. Many people find that a laxative works for a certain time – maybe weeks or months – but after that it seems to become ineffective. Once they try a different laxative, all is well again – for a while. This is because most laxatives are not supposed to be used for extended periods of time because people can develop a tolerance to them which means the medication will stop working. So it might take some time to find what works best. If you find you cannot comfortably have a bowel movement after taking laxatives for some time, talk to your GP.

Bulk-forming laxatives

As the name suggests, these laxatives work by increasing the volume of bulk going through the gut. Bran products, and products such as Ispaghula, are taken after a meal; they are not absorbed but pass through the gut, drawing in a large volume of water which makes it easier for the faeces to pass through the gut, and therefore easier to have a bowel movement.

Stimulant laxatives

Stimulant laxatives, as the name suggests, stimulate the gut, which speeds up the passage of waste matter through it, leaving less time for water to be absorbed. Thus faeces are more liquid, which makes it easier to have a bowel movement. These laxatives take around 10 hours to work. Ask your pharmacist to show you their range of stimulant laxatives, which may include products such as Dulcolax and Senokot.

Most remedies for constipation are not suitable for long-term use (these include the ones mentioned above). This is because they can cause an imbalance of fluids and salts and can lower potassium levels in your blood.

Osmotic laxatives

Osmotic laxatives increase the amount of fluid in the bowels; this fills up the bowels and thereby stimulates muscle contractions which move the faeces along the gut. A common osmotic laxative is Lactulose, which can be bought over the counter. You might experience some adverse effects when you first start taking osmotic laxatives; these are typically flatulence and stomach pains, but they should disappear as you continue the treatment. It might take a few days before the laxatives work properly. Magnesium citrate is also an osmotic laxative; this can be obtained from health stores or online retailers. However, magnesium can disturb the balance of electrolytes if taken too long and/or in large amounts. Electrolytes are minerals such as salt (sodium chloride) and magnesium (taken in through foods and drinks) between which the body works to maintain a healthy balance. If you take extra supplements – for example, magnesium – then the electrolyte balance can become disturbed and give you symptoms, such as abdominal pain.

However, a solution called polyethylene glycol electrolyte (PEG) is rapidly becoming the most frequently used osmotic laxative. This is because it is not absorbed into the body. It contains potassium, sodium and other minerals to replace electrolytes which are lost from the body during defecation. There are several names for this substance depending on which country you are in. In the UK this is called Movicol or Macrogol. In the US it is called Miralax or Glycolax.

Physical exercise and IBS symptoms

Time and time again in media reports we are told how important physical exercise is and how most people don't do enough of it, and indeed exercise is important in maintaining both physical and psychological health. However, the relationship between exercise and the gut isn't completely straightforward, as intense, strenuous exercise has been linked to a number of gastrointestinal symptoms, such as heartburn and diarrhoea[21]. Around 20–50% of endurance athletes experience these symptoms, although this is usually transient and does not develop into IBS. There is a lack of published research on the benefits of exercise in IBS but there is an increasing understanding of the effects of exercise on the GI system that we can consider. However, as with any major lifestyle change, if you want to start exercising and haven't done so before you should discuss this with your healthcare practitioner first and also introduce physical exercise gradually.

Constipation

A group of researchers from the Netherlands divided 43 physically inactive middle-aged people into two groups; one group simply carried on as they normally would (receiving standard treatment from their GPs) and the other group received a 12-week exercise programme. The people who were asked to exercise did 30 minutes of brisk walking and 11 minutes of home-based physical exercises a day. After three months of regular exercise, the men and women in this study saw improvements in three out of four of the criteria for constipation (percentage of incomplete defecations, percentage of defecations requiring straining and percentage of hard stools), which meant that fewer people had a diagnosis of constipation at the end of the research[22]. The time taken for food to be digested after eating and its waste excreted (known as 'transit time') also decreased in those who exercised regularly. Therefore, if you have IBS-C, you might want to consider a daily low or moderate level of exercise, such as a walk, swim or bike ride (if you're able to do these with your current IBS symptoms).

Diarrhoea

Although low or moderate amounts of exercise seem to be good for otherwise healthy people with constipation, strenuous exercise appears to trigger bouts of diarrhoea. You may have heard the term 'runners' trots', or remember long-distance runner Paula Radcliffe having to take an unscheduled stop in the 2005 London Marathon. Paula went on to win the race so this urgent attack didn't seem to hamper her progress too much but it was undoubtedly embarrassing and she must have been fed up with journalists asking her about it afterwards. This doesn't appear to happen when exercise is at a lower level and most people who run or jog moderately will never experience this type of exercise-induced diarrhoea.

Exercise and degree of IBS symptoms

One questionnaire study looked at whether women with IBS exercised more or less than those without the condition. In one study, more women without IBS exercised regularly (71%) than those who had IBS (48%). When just looking at the women with IBS, those who were more physically active were less likely to report incomplete evacuation after a bowel movement and less fatigue, although overall GI symptoms didn't seem to differ in women who did and those who did not exercise[23]. Even though this study is interesting, because it compared different people at one point in time rather than looking at symptoms before and after an intervention (such as an exercise programme), it's impossible to say whether the physical activity led to the promising findings or on the other hand, if having IBS led over time to the women doing less exercise. The latter would be understandable as exercise, particularly group exercise, may seem a terrifying prospect to someone with severe IBS symptoms. Nevertheless, this research does support some of the results from non-IBS studies in the sense that physical activity appears to help with constipation.

Other benefits of physical exercise

Physical activity has also been shown to protect against the development of colon cancer, gall stones and possibly inflammatory bowel disease[21]. Also, there is a huge amount of evidence that shows how regular exercise can help to lift our mood and increase general well-being. We certainly need some more specific studies to investigate the benefits, or otherwise, of physical activity in IBS so that specialist programmes can be created and integrated into care if positive results are found. However, if your primary IBS symptom is constipation, a 30-minute daily brisk walk could be something to include in your overall symptom-management strategy.

Tips for good quality sleep

In Chapter 2 we briefly explored the relationship between sleep quality and IBS. There are several 'sleep hygiene' recommendations that can help you to get a better night's sleep. These include:

- Avoid caffeine (in both foods containing chocolate and caffeinated drinks) and nicotine after 17:00, or midday if your sleep is particularly poor. Although decaffeinated drinks shouldn't keep you up at night, you may still want to skip decaf tea and coffee before bed as these can irritate the bladder or simply wake you up with the need to urinate. Also, as the bladder and bowel are closely related, irritation of one can impact on the other (many people with IBS also experience chronic bladder inflammation or interstitial cystitis).

- In addition to chemical stimulants found in coffee, tea, cigarettes, etc., steer clear of stimulation in the form of loud and lively television and music before bed. Many people read at bedtime in order to fall asleep, but if the book content is particularly poignant or upsetting it may prevent or disturb sleep; therefore it would be better to use relaxation techniques rather than reading just before bed to get sleepy.

- Don't use smartphones, tablets or laptops in bed – a recent large study of teenagers has found a link between the use of such devices and lack of sleep[24]. Scientists are starting to uncover the effect of the light from such screens on our circadian rhythm, or sleep–wake cycle, which seems to be telling our brains that it is daytime and we mustn't sleep.

- However, getting enough natural light during the day is important for good quality sleep. If you spend most of your time indoors during the day, try to use any breaks to expose yourself to natural daylight. It doesn't need to be sunny for your brain to recognise the daylight, so even going outside on an overcast day can help. This can also help to boost your vitamin D levels, which are important for overall health. In the dead of winter when daylight hours are at a minimum, you can buy natural light boxes. These come in many different shapes and sizes, so you can use them without it seeming like a chore; for instance there are natural-light desk lamps that can act as a normal desk light for working at the computer).

- Make sure that your bedroom is properly ventilated, either by keeping a window slightly open or, if you have vents in your window glazing, ensure that these are released. If your room is very stuffy in the summer a fan can help too.

- It is better for your body to cool down rather than need to warm up for sleep; therefore a warm bath at bedtime can help.

- Similarly, check that your bedroom is a good temperature for *you*. People vary in how hot/cold they need a room to be to sleep well so your requirements may differ from your partner's. If this is the case, it's important to discuss the temperature of the room and come to a compromise (perhaps one person may need to wear warmer pyjamas during winter, for example).

- Try to go to bed at a similar time each night as a regular bedtime routine can trigger sleepiness. Also, get up at the same time each day, even on weekends. Although it may seem logical that we can 'catch up' on lost sleep at the weekend, long lie-ins usually result in poorer sleep the next night and sometimes even head-aches and grogginess in the morning

- If you have any worries, write these concerns down before bed and 'park' them. It can help to set aside time each day (even just 10–15 minutes) to do this so that these niggles don't bubble up in your mind just as you get into bed.

It may take a little time to develop good quality sleep and sleeping habits; persist with the above advice for a number of weeks to give your body a chance to become accustomed to your new sleep routine. Sound sleep can benefit numerous areas of life so it is worth ditching the TV, smartphone and late-night chocolate. But bear in mind that everyone needs slightly different amounts of sleep – if you need more than your partner that's okay. If you feel fine on less sleep than your friends, don't worry and try to force yourself to sleep more; getting enough is important (quantity) but quality is also key to feeling refreshed.

Sleep restriction

If you've tried all the hints and tips above and are still having difficulties with your sleep, you may want to try a technique called 'sleep restriction'. During this method you drastically reduce your time in bed in an effort to re-set your body clock and increase your body's internal drive for sleep. Sleep restriction needs commitment for it to be successful, but the benefits can be better quality sleep, decreased fatigue and less daytime sleepiness.

Before you start reducing your time in bed, you must calculate your personal sleep efficiency. Sleep efficiency is the time you are asleep divided by the time you spend in bed at night (not including any daytime naps – these should be avoided when attempting sleep restriction) and then this figure is multiplied by 100 to give a percentage:

$$(\text{time asleep} \div \text{time in bed}) \times 100 = \% \text{ sleep efficiency}$$

People without sleep disorders, chronic illness and/or other health problems generally have a high level of sleep efficiency, for example:

$$(7.25 \text{ hrs} \div 8 \text{ hrs}) \times 100 = 91\% \text{ sleep efficiency}$$

However, if you have a condition that disturbs your sleep this can be much lower:

$$(5.5 \text{ hrs} \div 9 \text{ hrs}) \times 100 = 61\% \text{ sleep efficiency}$$

You can simply calculate your sleep efficiency by noting down the time you think you fell asleep and woke up, excluding any period of wakefulness in the night; but you can also use a smartphone app or sleep tracker. The latter is usually included in an activity-monitoring package, but these can be expensive so it's perfectly fine to calculate your sleep efficiency manually. These calculations need to be collected over a two-week period so that you can find out your average sleep efficiency, which will balance out any very bad (or good) nights. Simply add all the sleep efficiency percentages and divide by the number of nights (e.g. 14 for two weeks) and you'll have your average figure.

In the next stage of this technique, you need to decide a time to wake up which is suitable and natural for you and get up at this time for a week. This is important in order to start resetting your personal body clock so don't feel you need to set a time that's consistent with anyone else. If you naturally rise at 06:00 every day for a week then this is your wake time. For this reason, and because sleep restriction

can be taxing at first, you may want to do this at a time when you
have relatively few commitments (if this is possible).

Next, the restriction starts with you only spending the time in bed
that you're actually asleep. If we go back to the example above of
61% sleep efficiency where only 5.5 hours of the 9 hours spent in bed
was time asleep, here you would need to go to bed at 00:30. and set
your alarm for 06:00 so that you are in bed for only the same time
as you actually slept in the previous two weeks (5.5 hours). This may
feel quite hard at first if you've previously been going to bed at 21:00
(presumably because you're very tired and want to get some rest) so
you need to be disciplined at this stage. However, if you do find it's
just too difficult then adjust the time you set your alarm and go to
bed a little earlier - for example, go to bed at 23:30 and wake at 05:00.
But ideally, you should be getting up at your natural time.

You need to recalculate your sleep efficiency with this new restricted
time in bed. So, it may be on your first night of reduced time in bed:

(4 hrs ÷ 5.5 hrs) x 100 = 73% sleep efficiency

Even if you feel tired, the point here is that your sleep efficiency
increases from 61% to 73% and this is the start of a process that can
take several (usually six) weeks – it will get easier. If the percentage
does indeed increase, keep to this sleep schedule for one week. If
your sleep efficiency doesn't improve, reduce the amount of time
in bed for the next night to the amount of time you slept the night
before, meaning you'll be spending even less time in bed and going
to sleep later.

If you find that you sleep the entire 5.5 hours (or most of it) for a
full week, then the next stage is to increase your time in bed by 15
minutes, so go to bed at 00:15 and set the alarm for 06:00. Do this
for at least two weeks and calculate your sleep efficiency to make
sure you're sleeping for the increased amount of time. If your sleep

efficiency starts to dip again, reduce the time in bed back to the time slept once again for one week. However, if after a week you're sleeping for the increased time, you can add another increment of 15 minutes, or more if you wish. Do bear in mind though that the sleep restriction method is a gradual process so large jumps in time spent in bed may reduce your sleep efficiency and put you back to square one, which can be frustrating.

Once you have reached an adequate sleep efficiency percentage you should be sleeping most of the time you are in bed. There is no hard-and-fast rule here so if you have a chronic illness like IBS that can disturb your sleep you may not want to aim for percentages in the 90s. Nevertheless, increasing your sleep efficiency will enable you to get a better quality of sleep and reduce daytime tiredness which can lead to a more stable mood, better concentration and an improved ability to cope with the challenges of IBS.

Daily routine

As well as fostering a good sleep routine, setting a regular schedule can help you cope with the unpredictability of an illness like IBS. In addition to eating, waking up and going to bed at fixed times, it can be helpful to arrange other parts of your day with some consistency. IBS can feel like a rollercoaster and sometimes it may seem like everyday life is out of control, so by keeping an ordered timetable a sense of control can be regained. Of course this is not always possible, which is why flexibility should undoubtedly be central to every aspect of life. Think of your routine along the lines of 'fixed but flexible', like tree branches that bend with the wind but stay firmly attached to the tree trunk. For instance, you may have included a 30-minute walk in your day in order to exercise moderately but your symptoms flare up after breakfast (even if you have had your normal diet – sometimes there appears no rhyme or reason for flare-ups); if you need to skip the walk for a day don't worry too much or feel downhearted. But also don't give up on it. Similarly, if you want to go to a party this will probably mean you will eat foods you would not normally eat. These foods may increase your symptoms but trust that they will pass as you are doing so many positive things to manage your IBS.

Summary

This chapter has outlined medications that might alleviate the symptoms of IBS and some other recommendations that can help not only improve your IBS symptoms but also your overall health. Each person needs to test these medical treatments as IBS varies from person to person; there are no definitive treatment guidelines that will work immediately for everyone diagnosed with IBS. (This is often the case with long-term conditions.) Also, IBS can alter over time so you may need to tweak your treatment regime if you find your health starts to deteriorate. If this does happen, please do go back to your doctor and discuss the changes as these could be due to something other than IBS.

Chapter 5

Nutritional treatments, diet and probiotics

Similar to gaining a diagnosis, discovering if certain foods affect IBS symptoms can take a bit of time. Some dietary changes may work for one person but not the next and this is probably because IBS develops from different sets of factors in different people (see Chapter 9). This can be quite frustrating but there are some generally accepted guidelines for foods to avoid and those to increase. What is important is that food and dietary changes and supplementation can be useful strategies for tackling IBS.

We recommended you use the symptom and food diary described in Chapter 3 (page 50) when making any dietary or treatment changes so that you can pinpoint if something is making your symptoms worse, or if they're improving (note that you still need to include all the areas in the symptom diary like feelings and stressors as these may be triggering symptoms rather than particular foods).

IBS and diet

Many people diagnosed with IBS say that foods affect their symptoms, especially immediately following a meal. We now know a lot more about the reasons why this might be. A large part of this is due to the gut microbiota, which we talked about in Chapter 1 (and will explore more in Chapter 9). Diet has a huge influence on gut microbiota, which in turn has an effect on inflammation and IBS symptoms. Some people are convinced that they have food allergies or intolerances and this could very well be true (see Chapter 3 for food allergy testing). Certain foods (outlined later in this chapter) are well known to increase symptoms in some, but not all, people with IBS.

Food allergies

The symptoms that arise when you are allergic to foods may be different from the symptoms of hay fever, but the mechanisms underlying both are very similar. The immune systems of people with hay fever and food allergies identify pollen – or food – as harmful. This sets off a chain reaction, as described below. In both cases, histamine is produced.

(We mention hay fever because it has been found that people who are allergic to certain pollens are more likely also to develop food allergies.)

Sometimes food allergies begin in childhood, and disappear later. Adults can acquire food allergies too, although only a minority of adults have this problem. How does this happen? When you digest your food, your immune system decides whether the constituents of the food are safe, or whether they are not. The immune system doesn't always get it right! Sometimes it misidentifies foods that you have been eating all your life as suddenly harmful. The immune system then sets off a train of events that leads to histamines being produced and symptoms arising. For those with IBS, the symptoms will be gastrointestinal. Most food allergies are associated with an over production of immunoglobulin E (IgE) antibodies in reaction to certain foods. If a high level of these IgE antibodies aren't found, it is unlikely that you will be diagnosed as having a food allergy (see more about diagnostic tests for food allergies in Chapter 3).

Food intolerance and sensitivities

'I'm always conscious of my IBS, but working with it has become part of my routine and I don't let it hold me back. There are some foods that I miss eating but the effects are just not worth it. I love going out to eat but in the past I was often left feeling bloated and uncomfortable at the beginning of the meal. Now I've learnt what triggers my IBS I can choose something that I know will be okay; even though that wouldn't necessarily be my first choice I'm happy to be eating out with friends again.

'I've learnt that junk food is a real trigger for my IBS and pinpointing this has made a vast improvement to how frequently I'm experiencing symptoms.'

Kwilole

Most adults who believe they are allergic to certain foods are more likely to have food intolerances or sensitivities rather than true food allergy as above. That is, they realise that eating certain foods causes them symptoms, but skin prick or blood tests are negative. It has been found that around 20% of adults report food intolerances and sensitivities.

The elimination diet

'In terms of diet, I have cut some things out. It's been a process of elimination. Caffeine really aggravates things, so that's gone. Beer, thank God, seems fine, but wine and shorts are a no go. Oily fish (e.g. mackerel) is bad, as are prawns, sushi and seafood generally, so I'm avoiding those for now. Mayo is also bad. There are probably other things, I just haven't figured them out yet!'

Justin

Unlike allergies to certain foods, sensitivities and intolerances are much harder to diagnose. The most commonly recommended way to find out if you have a food intolerance is an exclusion, or 'elimination', diet – that is, cutting out certain types of food from your diet for three to four weeks and then slowly reintroducing these one by one to see if any of your IBS symptoms come back or worsen. The foods generally suggested to remove are:

- gluten-containing foods, such as wheat, corn, barley, and rye
- all dairy (milk, butter, yoghurt, cream, etc)
- soy and soy products, such as tofu
- eggs
- meats such as pork, beef and chicken
- beans/lentils; this includes peanuts and cashew nuts
- vegetables such as tomatoes, potatoes, aubergine and peppers (sometimes known as 'nightshade vegetables')
- citrus fruits
- nuts
- spices such as paprika, cayenne, chilli powder
- caffeinated drinks
- alcohol
- refined sugars
- ready-made condiments, such as tomato ketchup, relishes, chutneys, soy sauce (which also includes soy, of course), barbecue sauce, teriyaki sauce.

You may be wondering, what is left if you cut out all these foods? There are plenty of other foodstuffs you can eat during the exclusion part of this self-testing; these include:

- rice and rice flour, millet, quinoa, tapioca, buckwheat, potato flour
- dairy substitutes, such as rice milk
- fish, lamb, wild game, venison and duck
- pine nuts, flax seeds
- all vegetables except corn, brassicas (cabbage family) and nightshade vegetables (see above)
- olive oil
- non-citrus fruits
- filtered or distilled water and herbal teas
- natural sweeteners, such as stevia and blackstrap molasses if needed.

'It seems that certain foods trigger it more than others, especially white grains – bread, cakes, biscuits – and carbonated drinks. So I changed to a healthy diet including lots of fresh fruit, vegetables, rye bread and sometimes gluten-free goodies. This seems to help and the last bout of IBS I think I had in 2011–13 could also be related to the stress and deadlines of me finishing my Masters.'

Maria

But doing an exclusion diet isn't easy, especially the first few days, so it is worth getting prepared by buying the foods that you can eat in advance and looking up recipe ideas that contain these foods.

After you have been on this exclusion diet for three to four weeks, add one type of food back into your diet. You need to keep a detailed diary of the foods you add back into your diet and list any symptoms that occur (see the symptoms diary section in Chapter 3). New foods can be added every two days; make sure to eat the foodstuff at least twice a day in a quite large amount so that your body can tell you if it's problematic. If you reintroduce a food and aren't quite sure if it triggers symptoms, stop eating it again for a week before trying it again. Some other tips when embarking on an elimination diet are:

- If you normally drink a lot of caffeine, cut this down gradually or you may experience withdrawal symptoms

- When you reintroduce foods, make sure they are in a pure form rather than mixed into a recipe with other foodstuffs

- Even though you may lose weight during the elimination period, this is not a weight-loss diet so dropping pounds should not be the goal here

- If you do regular, strenuous exercise, consider cutting this down during the diet to avoid overly straining your body

- Try your best to get plenty of sleep and reduce stress during this time if possible. You may want to embark on this diet when you have some time off work (at least during the first few days)

- If you feel very low in energy, eat 'little and often' to prevent your blood sugar levels from dipping

- Most important, be patient. You may experience feelings of fatigue, headaches and/or muscle pain when you start this process as any major change in diet will trigger a type of withdrawal reaction. These symptoms should pass in a few days and often people feel much better on the diet, so stick with it!

Common food intolerances

Although an exclusion diet can be beneficial to find out which foods trigger symptoms for you, we do now know that for IBS certain foods seem more troublesome than others. For instance, researchers Gerard Mullin and colleagues in 2014 said that most intolerances in IBS result from carbohydrates[25]. They tested 15 people to see if reducing the amount of carbohydrates in the diet would help alleviate symptoms and found that all reported improvements in stool frequency and consistency, pain and quality of life. This confirmed other small studies where people following low-carbohydrate diets found it helped their symptoms.

Trigger foods

Although different foods may trigger symptoms in different people, here are some that are known particularly to aggravate IBS:

- carbohydrate-rich foods such as breads*, cakes and cereals

- spices

- dairy products

- legumes (beans and pulses)

- lentils

- chick peas

- gluten (wheat, barley and rye especially).

* Not all breads are baked the same way. Adele Costabile and colleagues at Reading University looked at the effect of the bread-making process on people with IBS[26]. They suggest that sourdough products may be best for these patients as this has a positive effect on the composition of the gut microbiota.

High histamine/fermented foods are also often problematic:

- alcohol

- pickles

- matured cheeses

- citrus fruits

- vinegar

- tomatoes

- legumes (beans and pulses)

You may want to try a stepped approach to an elimination diet by first eliminating these foods that are known culprits in IBS.

FODMAPs

Recently, there has been a great deal of interest in FODMAPs, which stands for: fermentable oligosaccharides, disaccharides, monosaccharides and polyols. These are sugars and carbohydrates which are not absorbed very well and are very quickly fermented by bacteria. Eating these foods to excess (a 'high FODMAP diet') can lead to an aggravation of IBS symptoms. Recent studies found that restricting fructose (the sugar found in fruit and corn) significantly improved IBS symptoms and that people on high FODMAP diets had worse symptoms than people on a low FODMAP diet. Jacqueline Barrett at the Monash University in Australia found that up to 86% improved on a low FODMAP diet [27]. Specific symptoms that were helped were bloating, wind, abdominal pain and altered bowel habits.

Examples of foods that contain high FODMAPs are:

- lactose : milk, dairy products, ice cream

- fructose:

- some fruits, such as mango, pear, apple
- some vegetables, such as asparagus, peas
- honey and syrups made from corn, maple, fruits
- sorbitol : some fruits, such as peaches, plums, apricots
- fructan:
  - some fruits, such as peaches, watermelon
  - some vegetables, such as artichokes, leeks
  - some grains, such as wheat, barley, rye
  - some nuts and legumes, such as pistachios and cashews.

Foods that are low-FODMAP include:

- lactose-free milk and yoghurts, rice milk, hard cheeses and sorbets
- fruits such as bananas, blueberries, grapefruit, grapes, honeydew melon, kiwifruit, citrus fruits (lemons, limes, mandarins, oranges)
- vegetables such as bamboo shoots, pak choi, carrots, celery, green beans, lettuce, parsnips, pumpkin.

We don't recommend you cut these high-FODMAP foods out without consulting a dietician or nutrition specialist as she will be able to assess your eating practices and lifestyle and give you a personalised eating plan. Alternatively, you can invest in a specialist book that gives you detailed information on the FODMAP approach.

Bacteria supplements

Some people with IBS have been found to have a reduction in the beneficial bacteria in the gut (*Lactobacilli* and *Bifidobacteria*). These have anti-inflammatory effects and it is now thought that some people with IBS have low-grade gut inflammation (this will be explored in detail in Chapter 9, page 143). So prebiotics and probiotics might help here.

'I take a multivitamin with pre- and probiotics, every day. They have really helped me and I would recommend that people try them.'

Robert

The difference between prebiotics and probiotics

Prebiotics

Prebiotics are supplements or substances in certain foods that nourish the beneficial bacteria already in the gut. They help digestion, absorption of nutrients and improve the immune system. In a recent study of 105 people with IBS who were given either the prebiotic fructan or a placebo (inert substance looking like the real prebiotic), it was found that there was a decrease in IBS symptoms in those who took the prebiotic. Another study found that taking a prebiotic supplement increased the number of bifidobacteria (good bacteria) in the gut, and improved bloating and stool consistency.

Prebiotics have been found to reduce the time it takes for waste matter to travel through the gut. However, they may also have unwanted effects, such as wind, in people who are prone to this.

Probiotics

Probiotics are live bacteria ingested in foods such as yoghurt and sauerkraut, and in probiotic supplements. They can help to populate the gut microbiota with good bacteria after someone has taken antibiotics, which wipe out all gut bacteria, good and bad. Researchers Rogha and colleagues in 2014 carried out a study on 85 people by giving them either a probiotic or a placebo[28]. They found that those who had the real probiotic experienced a reduction in abdominal pain and diarrhoea. Constipation was not affected. When researchers have looked at whether there are benefits to people with IBS by considering the results of a large number of studies together (called a 'meta-analysis'), it seems that probiotics are effective. Lactobacilli and bifidobacteria are the main constituents in probiotic supplements.

We recommend you take both pre- and probiotics together. Health stores sell these supplements together in one pot.

Gastroenterologists Fergus Shanahan and Eamonn Quigley recently wrote an article about the role of pre- and probiotics for the treatment of IBS and IBD. They cautioned that the effects are modest. They also said that in adults, *probiotics* do not remain in the gut and so have to be taken indefinitely for the effects to continue.

Probiotic yoghurts

Recently researchers investigated the usefulness of probiotic yoghurt. Altogether, 83 people with IBS consumed either the yoghurt or a placebo drink twice daily for six weeks. The research team found that the yoghurt helped with some symptoms of IBS and resulted in slight changes in some gut microbiota. In terms of IBS symptoms, the researchers found significant reductions in abdominal pain and other IBS symptoms.

Flavonoids

Flavonoids are substances that are synthesised by plants. These substances are beneficial to our health as they have antioxidant, antiviral and antibacterial properties. 'Flavanols' are one type of flavonoid.

Flavonols

Flavonols are naturally occurring substances in various foods that have antioxidant qualities. Such foods are good for us, as they help to lower the likelihood of developing diseases such as diabetes. It may therefore be worthwhile to include flavonol-rich foods in your diet (see below). However, we do not recommend that you take any flavonoid supplements. Although foodstuffs containing flavonoids are considered safe for us to consume, taking supplements is more risky as they might interact with other dietary flavonoids or medications. One study found that taking supplements might have a bad effect on the function of the thyroid. Ingesting lots of different flavonoid products might have side effects – we just don't know yet. So at the moment, the best thing is to eat a healthy diet that contains the flavonol-rich foods listed below.

- cocoa

- dark chocolate (70% cocoa at least)

- apples

- pomegranates

- red grapes

- tea

- red wine.

'I've been looking at foodstuffs which contain high flavonoids, as someone told me they can help your IBS as they are anti-inflammatory. My GP said it was a really good idea so I have lots of cocoa and black tea, and so far it has worked really well.'
Sarah

A note on cocoa

In 2011 a team from the Department of Food and Nutritional Sciences at the University of Reading carried out what is called a 'randomised control trial' – the most rigorous type of clinical research – to compare the gut microbiota of people who consumed a drink that was either low in cocoa flavonols (23 mg cocoa) or high in cocoa flavonols (494 mg cocoa)[29]. Cocoa beans have high levels of flavonols, although cocoa drinks differ in the amount of flavonols they contain. For the Reading team, they ensured that the cocoa they used had high levels. Altogether, 22 healthy people took part in the study, drinking the cocoa every evening for four weeks. After a four-week break, the people who had the low-cocoa drink then consumed the high-cocoa drink for four weeks and the people who had previously had the high-cocoa drink consumed the low-cocoa drink for four weeks.

This was a complicated and detailed study where participants were given various tests, such as measuring cholesterol and blood

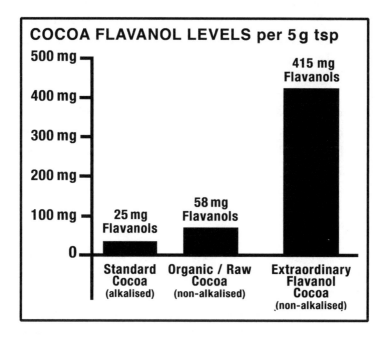

Figure 4 Bar chart showing the different levels of flavonol in different types of cocoa per 5 gram teaspoon. The bar on the right-hand side is a product called CHOCOCRU® which has exceptionally high levels of flavonol. (source: http://chococru.com, with permission)

pressure and giving blood and faecal samples. The team also measured the type and number of microbiota in the gut.

They found that compared with the low-cocoa drink, the high-cocoa drink increased the number of good bacteria (*Bifidobacteria* and *Lactobacilli*) and decreased the bad bacteria (clostridia). The authors concluded that drinking cocoa flavonols can positively affect gut microbiota. Different brands of cocoa differ in the amount of flavonols they contain. Most brands contain between 25 mg and 58 mg per teaspoon of cocoa. However, we have found a firm that sells cocoa products with much higher levels of flavonols called Chococru (http://chococru.com, see Figure 4). This chocolate also provides significant levels of iron and magnesium. There is no cholesterol in the cocoa, and it is fat-reduced. Most cocoas are 24% fat (from cocoa butter), whereas Chococru is 11–12%. Because this product is high in cocoa flavonols but low in fat, you shouldn't gain weight by eating it in moderation.

Cocoa flavonols also appear to help with memory problems later in life[30] and heart health[31]. But for IBS patients the most relevant aspect of cocoa flavonols is that they positively affect the microbiota in the gut, which is similar to the effects of prebiotics and probiotics – only they taste nicer!

Fibre

Studies show that ingesting fibre is important for healthy microbiota as this can protect against inflammation. The type of diet we have in the West, where foods are stored and processed, leads to a diet low in fibre. It is important to get enough fibre, not just to protect against IBS symptoms, but to reduce the likelihood of inflammation and ensure the microbiota are as diverse as possible as this helps in immune function. However, there are two types of fibre and it's important if you have IBS to know the distinction – soluble and insoluble. Soluble fibre dissolves in water and forms a gel-like substance which slows digestion and the rate at which we empty our stomach, whereas insoluble fibre has a laxative effect.

Foods containing soluble fibre:

- Oatmeal, oat cereal and oat bran

- Lentils and beans

- Fruits such as apples, strawberries, blueberries, oranges and pears

- Vegetables such as cucumbers, celery, carrots and dried peas

- Flaxseeds and chia

Foods containing insoluble fibre:

- Whole wheat flour, whole wheat bread, whole wheat cereal and wheat bran

- Whole grains, whole grain breads, whole grain cereals

- Barley, couscous, brown rice and bulgur wheat

- Vegetables such as courgettes, celery, broccoli, cabbage, onions, tomatoes, carrots, cucumbers, green beans, dark leafy vegetables

- Raisins and grapes

- Root vegetable skins.

NB: These lists aren't comprehensive – please see https://www.prebiotin.com/resources/fiber-content-of-foods/ which lists numerous foods and both their soluble and insoluble fibre content (this is an American site so it describes food portions in cups which equates to around 236 grams equivalent).

If you suffer from constipation, you may think it would be helpful to increase your portions of insoluble fibre but this is not necessarily the case. In a study of 275 people who had visited their GPs about IBS, those who were given soluble fibre in the form of psyllium (see below) improved over a 12-week period compared with people who were given insoluble fibre (bran) or a placebo food[32]. Insoluble fibre can have a powerful effect on the bowel; in fact in this study many patients dropped out of the trial as they couldn't tolerate the bran and their IBS symptoms worsened.

Because fibre is a common component of healthy foods like nuts, seeds, fruits and vegetables (and very important for overall health) the best approach to take for all types of IBS is to focus on the soluble types, such as oats. For fruits and vegetables high in insoluble fibre, the impact of their effect on the bowel can be lessened by peeling them, as much of the insoluble fibre is in the outer skins rather than the flesh. Chopping, cooking, and pureeing can also help, rather than simply eating raw vegetables, and fruits can be blended into a smoothie. Avoid eating insoluble fibre on an empty stomach (such as first thing in the morning) and also mix soluble and insoluble fibre at meal times with a larger proportion of soluble fibre foods.

However, if you or your healthcare practitioner feel that in addition to dietary changes you still need more fibre, you can also buy soluble fibre in the form of psyllium supplements in healthfood stores. Psyllium is a supplement made from the plantago ovata plant and has been shown to be beneficial in the management of IBS symptoms.

Other food and drinks worth trying

Peppermint, in the form of oil capsules, has been shown to reduce the symptoms of IBS and it is as effective as antispasmodics[32, 7]. These capsules can be prescribed by your GP or bought in a healthfood store. Peppermint tea can also help with stomach pain and spasms. Chamomile and fennel can also be used as antispasmodics.

There is also evidence that turmeric can be beneficial[33]. Turmeric is a traditional remedy for abdominal pain, indigestion, and bloating which can either be added in cooking or taken as a supplement.

Artichoke leaf in the form of an extract has been shown to reduce abdominal pain, cramps, bloating, flatulence, and constipation[33]. There are also countless products on the market with various combinations of herbs, the discussion of which is outside the scope of this book.

Dietary advice

General

- Eat oat-based products instead of wheat-based
- Eat linseeds every day – you may need to experiment with the dose, starting from a teaspoonful, up to a tablespoonful
- Drink pre- and probiotic yoghurts or take pre- and probiotic supplements.

Dietary advice for diarrhoea

- Limit the amount to caffeinated coffee and tea you drink and choose decaffeinated coffee, fruit and herbal teas, or decaffeinated tea.
- Eat soluble fibre-containing foods rather than foods high in insoluble fibre.

Dietary advice for constipation

In addition to the practical points given throughout this section the following two items will stand you in good stead:

- Eat oat-based products instead of wheat-based
- Drink water; coffee in moderation

Summary

We are learning more and more about the effects of certain foods and why they might be beneficial for people with IBS (and also the ones to avoid). Many foods are anti-inflammatory and some help balance our microbiota (gut bacteria). However, you may have certain food sensitivities or intolerances that need to be identified and dealt with in addition to the general guidance in this chapter. Overall, there is a great deal that can be done with dietary changes to improve your health and eliminate the symptoms of IBS.

In the next chapter we will be looking at some psychological and behavioural treatments that have been found to help.

Chapter 6

Psychological and behavioural approaches to managing IBS

This chapter looks at some psychological and behavioural ways to deal with some of the symptoms of IBS. In Chapter 1 we outlined how the brain and gut interact via the **brain–gut axis** (BGA; we'll explore this again in more detail in Chapter 9). Feeling like you have little control over your body and experiencing unpredictable embarrassing symptoms can cause a great deal of stress and anxiety. You may not have felt anxious or worried before your IBS started but now, like many invisible illnesses, the consequences of IBS may have resulted in a vicious cycle whereby feelings of loss of control feed back into the BGA and worsen symptoms. The types of therapies outlined in this chapter help to deal with the heightened feedback loop within the BGA, so tackling this should help to reduce IBS symptoms. Hence these types of therapies can be important additions to your treatment package.

Clinical hypnosis and gut-directed hypnotherapy

Clinical hypnosis, or hypnotherapy, is an increasingly common and well-evidenced type of therapeutic technique used in many conditions, including asthma, headaches and migraine, chronic pain in cancer patients and IBS. In fact, hypnotherapy is one of the most researched types of treatment for managing the symptoms of IBS at present.

How does hypnotherapy work?

A modern-day clinical hypnotist or hypnotherapist aims to bring about a state of suggestibility, known as a 'hypnotic state', by using exercises that induce deep relaxation. The idea of a hypnotic state may sound a bit strange and unnatural, but it is simply an altered state of awareness, a bit like daydreaming. For instance, have you ever been doing an everyday activity, such as having a shower, but because you have been thinking about something else (perhaps work that you need to do) you can't remember if you've washed your hair? You then check your hair and you have indeed washed it but simply don't remember as your awareness was somewhere else. Hence, altered awareness is a daily occurrence and causes us no significant problems at all.

Within hypnotherapy, the therapist will help you to reach a hypnotic state wherein the mind is more open to the process of change. The therapist will then make suggestions that can help with a range of issues, including the symptoms of IBS. There are two main methods for using hypnotherapeutic techniques in IBS; these are called the 'Manchester Approach' and the 'North Carolina Protocol', which have been researched and shown to be effective.

The Manchester Approach to hypnotherapy in IBS

The Manchester Approach was the first type of hypnotherapy to be properly studied and reported on in the medical and scientific community. Professor Peter Whorwell and his colleagues at the University of Manchester published their seminal paper in the esteemed journal the *Lancet* in 1984, which showed that patients who had been treated with hypnotherapy had much better outcomes in terms of abdominal pain, abdominal distension, bowel habit and general well-being in comparison to patients treated with psychotherapy. These beneficial changes were seen to last when the patients were tested again three months after the therapies finished[34].

Over the years, Professor Whorwell and colleagues have further developed this technique into what is now known as the Manchester Approach. With this method, the therapist will first take a detailed personal and medical history, talk the patient through reasons why they may have IBS symptoms and how the therapy work and also reassure the patient throughout. This protocol now consists of 12 sessions, although when Professor Whorwell first started with this technique it was only seven[35].

After the patient history has been taken and the method explained, the first couple of sessions are used to allow patients to get used to the process of hypnotherapy. A hypnotic state is reached by progressive physical relaxation (tensing and relaxing muscles sequentially throughout the body from the toes to the fingers) and exercises such as repeating the word 'calm' on the out breath. General exercises to increase well-being are used also – for example, metaphors that bring to mind a sense of calm and relaxation, such as sinking into a soft cushion or cloud, being on holiday somewhere in the warm sunshine or the gentle rocking of a tethered boat.

Next come the 'gut-directed' sessions. These start in the same way as the general hypnotherapy sessions, by inducing a hypnotic state, but the exercises focus on the gut. For instance, a patient will be asked to create a picture in his/her mind of his/her gut when symptoms of IBS are flaring and then be directed by the therapist to calm it. This needn't be a literal image and could be something like a roller-coaster where the feelings of urgency are symbolised by the breakneck speed and twists and turns of the ride which, through the hypnotherapy, will metamorphose into a quiet, sedate country drive. Other types of gut-directed exercises include patients placing their hand on their abdomen and using the feeling of warmth as a sense of control over the stomach and its goings-on.

The final, but equally important, part of the Manchester Approach involves sessions that focus on reducing the fear and avoidance of situations that people with IBS might find difficult, such as a crowded train journey. Here, the therapist guides the patient through such a situation, but his/her symptoms are not triggered; rather, the gut remains calm, under control and not of concern.

At the end of the therapy patients are given a recording of the sessions so that the gut-directed hypnotherapy exercises can be practised at home. Hypnotherapy is like any other skill and so it must be practised to work well; patients are generally encouraged to use the tools taught to them on a daily basis. For details of how to find a hypnotherapist please see the end of this section (page 94).

The North Carolina Protocol for hypnotherapy in IBS

The North Carolina Protocol was developed by the clinical psychologists Drs Olafur Palsson and William Whitehead at the University of North Carolina at Chapel Hill, USA. This method differs somewhat from the Manchester Approach as it has standardised scripts that therapists work from, thus each patient receives the same information regardless of which therapist they consult. By developing a standard treatment 'package' Drs Palsson and Whitehead have simplified its delivery, making it easier to train therapists throughout the USA and beyond. This has also made researching the protocol easier as researchers know that every patient receives exactly the same input.

Patients have seven 45-minute sessions of clinical hypnosis over 12 weeks. The sessions are arranged in treatment modules that can be interchanged, depending on the patient's needs. Within these modules are five separate therapeutic components:

1. altering attention so that the patient can move away from 'tuning into' bowel sensations and symptoms

2. changing the perceptions the patient has of his/her symptoms

3. working on a sense of control, not only over IBS but general health and safety/comfort

4. hypnotic suggestions for the bowel to become immune to stress, upset and distressing life events

5. hypnotic suggestions and imagery which encourage normal and healthy GI function.

Therapists using the North Carolina Protocol have a set of tools that include a number of techniques. Eye fixation induction is one technique where the therapist will ask patients to fix their gaze on a set point, for instance the ceiling or the hypnotherapist's pen. This staring will tire the eyes and the therapist will also suggest that the patient's eyelids are becoming heavier and heavier so that eventually they close – once this occurs the patient is believed to be in a 'hypnotic state' or 'trance'. Next, the therapist will deepen the hypnotic state by guided systematic physical relaxation, or relaxation using scenes and imagery. Here, therapeutic suggestions can be made as the mind should be more open to change. The final process is trance termination, where the hypnotherapist gently and gradually brings the patient out of the hypnotic state, often by counting and giving suggestions of returning to full awareness. Dr Palsson and his team have carried out a number of research studies that show that this method of hypnotherapy, designed specifically for people with IBS, is beneficial – more than 80% of people in the research studies saw improvements in their condition following the treatment[36].

What does hypnotherapy feel like?

'Contrary to common belief, under hypnosis, the client is actually given back control of unwanted thoughts and behaviours. The so-called hypnotic "trance" is in reality just an enhanced state of concentration and relaxation.'

Ian Jackson, hypnotherapist

'Hypnosis', 'altered awareness', 'trance', etc may sound a little odd; however, it's important to bear in mind that you are still in control of your body and mind when engaging in hypnotherapy and if you do feel uncomfortable at any time, you can ask the therapist to stop and she will end the treatment. But most people enjoy the experience of deep relaxation, although you don't have to be relaxed to get the benefits of clinical hypnosis. Some people say they feel a sense of floating, whilst others may feel that their bodies are very heavy.

The type of hypnotherapy used to treat IBS doesn't involve the in-depth exploration of secrets or trauma – modern day gut-directed hypnotherapy is nothing like the Freudian idea of therapy. However, as IBS can feel like an embarrassing illness you may feel a little awkward when discussing symptoms and sensations; remember that a trained therapist will be entirely used to this and will not judge you in any way.

Is hypnotherapy safe?

The answer to this is quite simply, yes. A large number of research studies have demonstrated that hypnotherapy is safe and doesn't have the same type of side effects that some medications can have. Nevertheless, as with any other type of treatment or therapy, it is important that you find a practitioner who is appropriately trained. In the UK, hypnotherapy isn't a regulated profession so there aren't laws regarding the minimum level of qualifications and training that a person needs to have to call themselves a 'hypnotherapist'. This can make it difficult for patients to find the best therapist but there are professional bodies that 'self-regulate' in the UK. These organisations do have a set of standards that practitioners need to meet to be held on their lists and registers. There are quite a few of these self-regulatory bodies in the UK at present and it is a matter of opinion if one is better than another. Therefore, if you're looking for a hypnotherapist there's a very useful search tool on the Hypnotherapy Directory website (http://www.hypnotherapy-directory.org.uk/adv-search.html). Within this advanced search tool you can select 'Member of a professional body' which will only give you the results for therapists who have been vetted by a professional organisation. There is more information regarding the professional bodies that self-regulate hypnotherapy and also more general information on this type of treatment on the website.

Your GP may be able to refer you for hypnotherapy as the National Institute for Health and Care Excellence (NICE) recommends this as a treatment for IBS. But if you've found your GP to be less than supportive or the services are not offered by the NHS in your area, you might want to contact private practitioners yourself. If you do, it is worth asking some questions in addition to checking their qualifications and registrations with professional bodies, such as:

- How many people have you treated with IBS?

- Do you have any data on average success rates/benefits/symptom reduction?

- What type of hypnotherapy do you use for IBS?

- How many sessions would you recommend? (The therapist may not be able to answer this until after an initial consultation if he is not using a standard method.)

- What are the costs and cancellation policies? (A general hypnotherapy session is usually between £50 and £90 and most therapists would require a 24-hour notice of cancellation.)

- Do you offer low-cost sessions or concessionary rates for people on low incomes, such as students/retired/those on benefits (if appropriate)?

- Can I speak to someone with IBS who has been helped by you?

You may want to approach a few different therapists and see if you feel you like them after speaking on the phone, before making a booking.

Cognitive behavioural therapy

Cognitive behavioural therapy, or CBT, is a talking therapy that has been researched in a wide range of conditions, from depression and anxiety disorders to chronic pain and fatigue in cancer patients. This type of treatment is very structured with a problem-focused approach, as opposed to other forms of talking therapies that are more exploratory (e.g. psychotherapy). CBT is most commonly delivered by a trained and qualified therapist, but there are now many self-help books on the technique.

How does CBT work?

CBT works by helping you think closely about your thoughts and feelings and seeing how these influence your behaviour, which in turn loops back to how we feel and think about situations and experiences. It may seem obvious that our thoughts ('cognitions') affect our behaviours and vice versa, but we can all get caught in vicious circles. Over-thinking and ruminating on events, the future and even bodily sensations can impact on our hypothalamus–pituitary–adrenal (HPA) axis, and as we've seen in Chapter 1 (page 13), the HPA axis and brain–gut axis (BGA) link our digestive systems to our brains/cognitions/feelings (more about this in Chapter 9).

Although there are no standardised protocols for CBT in IBS, like the methods mentioned previously within hypnotherapy, there are common components that most CBT therapists will use with someone who has IBS. These are:

- Education/teaching on the relationship between stress and IBS symptoms (similar to the information in Chapter 9)

- Approaches to deal with life stresses that contribute to IBS symptoms

- Monitoring of IBS flare-ups and what happens before and after these symptom clusters

- Relaxation exercises (sometimes progressive physical relaxation of muscles but these can also be breathing exercises and imagery) to lower physiological arousal of the HPA axis and increase the sense of control over bodily activity

- 'Cognitive restructuring', which means changing the way we think about the world around us, as sometimes these patterns can play into our stress responses and in turn symptoms (see the next chapter for examples).

In a CBT session, the therapist will work through some exercises that challenge your thoughts and beliefs. You will most likely be given some 'homework' to do between sessions as well as it can take time and practice to change the way we think.

CBT requires quite a lot of work on the part of the patient; it is an active therapy rather than a passive treatment, such as taking medicines. You'll be asked to record your thoughts and feelings as well as your symptoms to see if you can identify links between them. Then you may be asked to try activities or foods that you felt were damaging or triggers for symptom flares and monitor what happens in order to identify and then change your reactions, which should help to dampen down the stress response and disengage an overactive HPA and BGA function.

Research into CBT for the treatment of IBS

Like hypnotherapy, IBS-specific CBT has been studied by many different research groups in numerous countries. Early studies showed promising results; for instance in a study with 20 IBS patients who either had intensive individual CBT or were asked to monitor their GI symptoms, 80% of the people who received CBT had improvements in their conditions whereas only 10% of those who symptom-monitored did[37]. Other studies compared CBT with standard medical care and similar benefits of CBT were found. However, these types of comparison groups weren't particularly similar as patients allocated CBT clearly had more time with practitioners and care than those who were not assigned to this group. Therefore, further studies split the patients into groups who received CBT and an intervention that gave people the same amount of human interaction, in this case a self-help support group. CBT still seemed a good option as 67% of people in this group said they had a reduction in GI symptoms, whereas only 31% of those in the self-help support group saw their symptoms improve. (There was also a symptom-monitoring group in which 10% of people reported a decline in symptoms.)[38] Further studies have shown more mixed results but overall it does seem that CBT can help to deal with some of the symptoms of IBS and also the anxiety and depression that can come with having an unpredictable and embarrassing illness[39].

Group CBT

CBT is a very popular treatment at present for many illnesses; this has led to researchers and medics developing novel ways to make this therapy available to more people. One such method that has been studied by researchers is group CBT which has the obvious benefit of reducing costs and potentially making it easier for healthcare providers to fund. A large study of 210 patients either had CBT or 'psychoeducational support' in a group of three to six people for 10 weeks. (Each session was 90 minutes long.) There was also a symptom-monitoring group to act as a comparison. If you're wondering what psychoeducational support means, in this study the group of patients given this treatment had a number of therapist-led discussions on IBS-related topics such as diet, food sensitivities, types of diagnostic tests and interactions with doctors. The key here was that the patients were encouraged to talk about their experiences with others who had the same condition and no standard therapeutic exercises took place, hence it was a bit like a support group but with specific areas of conversation. Interestingly, the researchers found improvements in peoples' IBS symptoms in *both* the CBT group and psychoeducational support groups, but not the symptom-monitoring group[40]. This is noteworthy in a couple of ways – first, that group CBT seems to be effective and so is yet another option for IBS patients, and, secondly, that simply discussing problems and illness experiences appears to help manage IBS symptoms. In Chapter 2 we touched on the effects of the hormone oxytocin in the context of supportive relationships, and how this can reduce the stress response and benefit our BGA/ HPA systems, so it's possible that support groups, even without any traditional therapeutic exercises, could be a therapy in themselves (see Chapter 7 for more on support groups).

Self-help CBT

Self-help CBT has also been investigated. There are lots of books on CBT available now and some specifically for people with IBS. Therefore, researchers interested in IBS, and particularly using CBT to treat IBS, conducted a scientific evaluation of a self-help book[41]. Although the number of people in this study was small (28 in total), it was found that after reading the self-help book and using the advice given, general GI symptoms declined, abdominal pain was reduced and perceptions of health and well-being improved[42]. Of course this was only a small study but it does illustrate the potential benefits of self-help books.

How do I find a CBT therapist?

There are a variety of professionals that may be trained in CBT – clinical and counselling psychologists, counsellors, CBT therapists, to name a few. Psychologists, whether from a clinical, counselling or health background, are trained to a high level and should have 'chartered status' with the British Psychological Society (BPS). The BPS is a representative body for psychologists in the UK. To become a chartered psychologist an individual needs to have completed a minimum of six years' education and training on BPS-recognised courses to doctorate standard. To find a chartered psychologist in your area who offers CBT you can use the BPS's directory (http://www.bps.org.uk/bpslegacy/dcp). Make sure you type in 'CBT' in the 'Additional Information' tab at the bottom of the page and you should receive a number of psychologists in your local area who offer this therapy. Once you've done this it is worth also checking that the psychologist is a 'practitioner psychologist', which means she has trained specifically to deliver therapy rather than, or in addition to, conducting research or work in other fields, such as policy-making.

Practitioner psychologists are regulated by the Health and Care Professions Council (HCPC; http://www.hcpc-uk.org.uk). The HCPC defines certain criteria in terms of professional skills, education and behaviour in order to protect members of the public. For instance, if a practitioner doesn't meet the HCPC's standards it can prevent her from practising. Patients can make complaints about psychologists to the HCPC, which will act upon the information. It's exactly the same sort of body as the General Medical Council that regulates doctors, so there is an avenue of recourse if anything should go awry within therapy. The title 'practitioner psychologist' is protected by law and anyone using this label without being registered with the HCPC can be prosecuted. You can check if someone is registered with the HCPC by searching his/her last name or registration number if you have it (http://www.hcpc-uk.org/check/). But remember, this is only for 'practitioner psychologists' – if someone simply says they're a therapist they probably won't be a member of the HCPC and potentially won't have been through the rigorous training that the HCPC requires.

Nevertheless, there are other professionals, such as counsellors and psychotherapists, who are trained to deliver CBT. The British Association for Behavioural and Cognitive Psychotherapies (BABCP) also has a register where you can find out if a therapist has completed an accredited CBT course and also locate CBT therapists in your area (http://www.cbtregisteruk.com/Default.aspx). As this register includes other types of professionals who are trained in CBT but are not psychologists, such as doctors, social workers and occupational therapists, you may want to contact the individual or look at her website to see exactly what type of patient she works with. (Unfortunately there isn't an easy way to search for this on the BABCP website.)

Mindfulness and meditation

The practice of mindfulness has become increasingly popular in recent years. Mindfulness is a particular form of meditation, stemming from Buddhism but now used in a secular fashion as a way to manage both stress and a number of illnesses, including chronic pain, anxiety and depression, stress in cancer patients and fibromyalgia. There are many different strands of mindfulness, including therapies that merge this technique with CBT (mindfulness-based cognitive therapy or MBCT) and specific stress-targeted strategies (mindfulness-based stress reduction or MBSR). Mindfulness techniques can also be part of a therapy called 'acceptance and commitment therapy' (ACT), which is a therapy that helps people to accept what they cannot change whilst equally committing to tackling areas in which quality of life can be improved. The common core of the mindfulness approach in all these therapies is the practice of bringing our attention to the moment, rather than mulling over the past or worrying about the future. A variety of meditative exercises are used to focus attention on the here and now, which we will explore more in Chapter 7 (page 114).

How does mindfulness work?

We tend to spend most of our lives on automatic pilot, rarely noticing what's happening in each moment. But on the flip side we do have the capacity to control our attention and focus on specific aspects of the environment and our internal sensations (such as mentioned previously in the hypnotherapy section). The basic tenet of mindfulness is that by zooming in on the present and becoming active, but non-judgemental, observers we can enrich our lives. This enrichment stems from the development of a greater sense of control over life, rather than the constant reactivity that we can become stuck in if we live too much in the past or future. Like the other treatments in this chapter, mindfulness does not claim to be a 'cure' for any condition, but rather it aims to enhance coping with the day-to-day effects of a chronic illness and the stresses that this inevitably places on a person. Also, this technique can help us to view ill health and 'wellness' as not mutually exclusive, instead helping us to realise that symptoms and health complaints are a natural part of life and life can still be enjoyable and fulfilling.

What are mindfulness exercises like?

Mindfulness exercises can be taught either on a one-to-one basis or in groups. The more structured treatments, such as MBSR, usually consist of eight to 10 weekly 2.5-hour sessions and can be delivered in large groups of up to 30 people at a time. Some courses also have a weekend day session, although there is wide variation in less structured courses. Typical components of MBSR are:

- meditation practice

- breathing techniques

- using mindfulness with gentle yoga/stretching postures

- mindfulness practice for ordinary activities, such as walking, standing, eating, etc.

- mindfulness techniques to use in stressful situations and social interactions.

(See Chapter 7 for examples of the above that you can practise at home.)

When using all of these techniques, individuals are instructed to sharpen their focus onto the observation target – this may be their breathing or merely the sensation of sitting on a chair. Numerous cognitions (thoughts) will drift into our minds when we try this – ideas, memories, daydreams, for example. To engage in mindful awareness, it's essential to note in your mind the nature of the cognition, without assigning any type of judgement or deep evaluation to it. Next, attention should be calmly pulled back to the moment and to the observation target, such as the sensation of your back resting against the chair. It's quite common to have thoughts that are judgemental in their nature when first practising mindfulness, such as 'Why on earth am I doing this, it's ridiculous and not going to help me'; even these types of thought should be noticed without judgement, perhaps simply categorised as 'a thought', nothing more, nothing less. Other types of information will pass through your mind, such as a police siren – this can be noted and labelled 'a noise' before gently moving your attention back to the mindfulness task. You may have an itch on your nose that can be logged as 'a physical sensation' and then, again, attention should be brought back to the mindfulness exercise. The purpose is to help you appreciate that most thoughts, feelings and sensations are transient and we need not become fixed within them.

People who attend MBSR classes are asked to practise the taught exercises for 45 minutes every day. This is because mindfulness is a skill and like any other skill it needs to be practised for someone to be able to access it when needed – for example, in a stressful situation such as an important meeting where it would be frowned upon to leave the room and use the toilet. Like the other therapies and techniques mentioned in this chapter, it is believed that mindfulness can influence the HPA axis and so help manage the symptoms of IBS by regulating the BGA /HPA function. Research has also shown that mindfulness can positively impact immune function[43], which could also benefit people with IBS.

Research into mindfulness techniques for IBS

Research into mindfulness techniques for IBS is a new field but it is gaining momentum. In a study of 75 women with IBS, each woman either attended training in mindfulness or a support group for eight weeks, with a final half-day session at the end of the courses. IBS symptoms were reported before and immediately after the mindfulness training and support group sessions, and after a further three months. Right after the courses, IBS symptoms decreased by on average 26% in those who engaged in mindfulness practice and only 6% in the support group. At three months, patients who had been taught mindfulness further improved with an average 38% reduction in symptoms compared with 11% in the support group[44]. Hence, learning, and using, the mindfulness techniques was more beneficial to the women in this study than social support alone.

Another study that included 90 patients with IBS (this time both men and women) found greater improvements in IBS symptoms following mindfulness training as compared with patients receiving standard treatment; 50% of people using the mindfulness techniques improved compared with 21% of those simply adhering to general advice from their doctors[45]. Therefore, evidence is gathering to support the use of mindfulness techniques for the management of IBS, although more work needs to be done to gain a comprehensive picture of exactly why mindfulness could help.

If you'd like to try a mindfulness approach, follow the guidance earlier in the chapter for accessing psychologists and counsellors in the previous section but ask specifically if the therapist has been trained in mindfulness techniques – an experienced professional should have a battery of methods she can use for a particular problem or condition and will be able to tailor therapy to your individual needs.

Internet mindfulness therapy

You don't have to see a therapist face to face, however, to try mindfulness techniques specifically designed for people with IBS. Brjánn Ljótsson and colleagues in Sweden have done a great deal of work on creating and evaluating an online programme that uses mindfulness exercises to help IBS patients accept the condition, rather than control it[46]. This approach may help people who do not find traditional CBT beneficial, although it does integrate CBT ideas into the mindfulness techniques. The mindfulness exercises included in this online programme were designed specifically to help people with IBS deal with the anxiety that can develop around IBS symptoms and how this anxiousness can lead to avoidance of certain situations or activities. This 10-week programme is divided into five steps, starting with an explanation of the treatment and mindfulness instructions. Steps 2, 3 and 4 build on the first step with a description of the theory behind the programme and continued advice on mindfulness techniques. The fifth and final step involves 'exposure exercises', in other words purposely triggering symptoms. This can be done by eating trigger foods, engaging in strenuous physical activity or by entering into a stressful situation. This may sound crazy but the point of this part of the programme is to use the mindfulness strategies when symptoms occur so that you can become less fearful of these situations. By reducing anxiety and avoidance, IBS symptoms can also decrease, which will lead to a better quality of life. Indeed, this is exactly what the researchers found when they compared this programme with an online discussion forum of 86 people where 42% of those who completed the mindfulness training saw improvements in their IBS symptoms[47]. Anxiety and depression also improved for the people using the mindfulness techniques, as did overall functioning.

Summary

This chapter has explored a number of psychological and behavioural techniques that can help people cope with an illness like IBS and potentially dampen the overactive BGA/HPA function that was briefly discussed in Chapter 1 and is looked at in more detail in Chapter 9. Whilst none of these methods claims to be curative, they have been shown in research studies to be beneficial to people with IBS. You may want to try one or more of these techniques alone or in addition to dietary changes and medication as they are not harmful and the potential benefits could indeed spill over to other areas of your life, promoting general well-being and quality of life.

In the following chapter we will outline various techniques that you can try yourself that can also help to reduce stress and worry and deal with the difficulties of living with IBS.

Chapter 7

Self-help strategies

'Living with the IBS dented my confidence quite a lot. I was scared of going places in case I got an attack. My symptoms got markedly worse at university and I got really angry that it was affecting my life so much. I was constantly embarrassed when trying to deal with my symptoms. Now, I'm completely open about it and have no problem just getting on with it. Don't get me wrong, having an attack when having a nice restaurant meal or day out still gets me down, but whereas it used to ruin my day and usually end up with me going home early, it is now just an annoyance that needs to be dealt with.'

Emily

In Chapters 4–6 we looked at various types of treatments that may help to manage the symptoms and effects of IBS. These mostly require consultations with professionals such as doctors, nutritional therapists and psychologists; however, there are many strategies you can try for yourself at home and at no cost. Many of the topics we discuss in this chapter are also good for general health, not just for dealing with IBS.

Dealing with stress and anxiety-provoking situations

In the previous chapter we talked about psychological and behavioural techniques, such as hypnotherapy, CBT and mindfulness, that can provide strategies to deal with the stress of having IBS. Whilst it can be nice to have professional guidance when you're learning these techniques, if you can't find a practitioner in your area, are on a tight budget or simply would rather not see a professional, some of the elements of these methods can be self-taught.

Cognitive strategies

There are certain ways of thinking that can negatively affect the way we view the world and ultimately our health, especially if someone has a condition like IBS that can be difficult to cope with at times.

> 'Impact on my life – initially it was huge. I wouldn't go places and regularly turned down invites for fear of having an attack. Work was a nightmare too. I'm sure part of it was a self-perpetuating cycle though, with concern about having an attack often bringing it on. Sadly, it affected my enjoyment of the social side of university quite a lot. I still find this quite upsetting, as I really feel like I missed out.'
>
> *Emily*

Catastrophising

Put simply, catastrophising is when we think the worst will happen and we have no control over a certain situation. An example of this might be, 'If I go to that concert and need the toilet there will be a big queue and I won't be able to control my bowels so I will have an accident and everyone will see and smell it and I'll never be able to go out in public again'. Although academics and psychologists may say this type of feeling is irrational, it won't seem to be unfounded to someone with IBS. The problem with catastrophising is that it can make us feel anxious even before we've left the front door! This anxiety or fear will play into the BGA/HPA function that we discussed in Chapter 1 (there will be more on this in Chapter 9) so by tackling this type of cognition (way of thinking), it is possible to reduce the stress-related aspects of IBS.

The first step in dealing with catastrophising is to acknowledge its existence – you don't know that the embarrassing situation will occur, you're imagining that it could, therefore it is not a foregone conclusion that if you attend a concert you will defecate in public. Next, if you feel your heart is pounding and you're breathing rapidly try one of the breathing exercises shown on pages 113–4 to kickstart your body's parasympathetic nervous system activity. The parasympathetic nervous system is an automatic, subconscious part of the central nervous system (CNS; see Chapter 1), which brings the body back into a stable, resting state after a fight-or-flight (stress) response. Finally, challenge your cognitions/thought patterns by playing the 'what-if' game:

- 'What if I go to a concert?' – You can practise the breathing and relaxation exercises in this chapter to help keep calm; avoid your trigger foods a few days before the event and on the day of the event; tell the person you're going with about your IBS and that you might need to find a toilet quickly; book seats near the aisle so you can exit easily.

- 'What if I need the toilet and there's a queue?' – Identify the disabled toilets before getting to the venue; go to the toilet just before the intermission to avoid the queues or carry a 'Can't Wait Card'. This is a small, wallet-sized card that is available through the IBS Network and can be used to access toilets urgently (http://www.theibsnetwork.org/what-we-offer/cant-wait-card). There is a travel version also which includes the 'can't wait' message in a vast number of languages.

- 'What if I can't control my bowels and I have an accident?' – Prepare an emergency pack (below).

- 'Everyone will see it and smell it and I'll never be able to go out in public again.' – In the unlikely event that you did have an accident, you'll have your emergency pack so you'll be able to deal with it quickly; you will not be trapped inside the concert venue so you can leave whenever you want/need to; you'll almost definitely never see these people again and anyway, does it matter what strangers think? Your IBS doesn't define you and does not make you a less valuable person; you're a strong individual to be coping with such an unpleasant condition.

To summarise, there are active things you can do before, during and after an event that will make it easier for you to cope with if symptoms occur. But chances are if you put all these strategies in place, they won't be needed as you'll feel more comfortable about going out and your BGA/HPA won't be in overdrive.

Finally, think about what's most likely to happen – 'I may have some IBS symptoms but because I've been using self-help strategies and prepared myself I will be able to deal with any symptoms and enjoy the concert.'

> 'My advice is to try to worry about it less and remember that in any awkward moments no-one else is anywhere near as bothered as you are. When I stopped worrying was when this really changed for me. I am not saying that I don't still get stressed. I still worry about stupid things and have emotional outbursts and I still get IBS attacks that upset me sometimes. What is different now is that these things feature in my life, rather than rule it.'
>
> *Emily*

Breathing techniques

We need different amounts of oxygen for different tasks. For example, when exercising our muscles will need more oxygen so breathing rates increase. We will also produce more carbon dioxide when breathing heavily like this. However, sometimes during a flash of panic or anxiety (for instance, at the first signs of a bout of diarrhoea) breathing rates quicken but, as our muscles will not be working any harder than when at rest, the extra oxygen taken in is not used and turned into carbon dioxide; as we will still be breathing out carbon dioxide at a faster rate than usual, this leads to lower-than-normal levels of carbon dioxide in our blood. This condition is known as 'respiratory alkalosis' and can lead to unpleasant sensations, such as pins and needles, or feeling clammy and sweaty and light-headed. This is generally a temporary condition as our pH levels will return to normal once we calm down. However, we can turn the situation around more quickly by noticing when our breathing quickens or changes and using exercises to kick-start the parasympathetic nervous system.

Breathing exercises can form part of your general relaxation programme to help manage the stress and anxiety associated with having IBS and they can also help in acute situations, such as an attack of symptoms when out and about. This is because breathing techniques can help stimulate the parasympathetic nervous system (as above) which will not only help to regulate the BGA/HPA but also make us feel calmer and more relaxed. If you think about it, how we breathe is strongly related to how we're feeling; if we've been startled by, say, a car coming out of nowhere which makes us brake suddenly whilst driving, our breathing will be rapid and shallow. But if we're at home relaxing, maybe reading a book, our breathing will most likely be slow and regular.

Below is an easy breathing exercise that you can try in everyday life to feel more focused and relaxed and it can also be used if you become anxious at the first signs of IBS flare-ups.

Simple breathing exercise

- Sit or lie down, in a comfortable place if possible (although it's fine to do this when standing if you need to).

- Close your eyes if desired, but if this makes you feel dizzy or unsteady then keep your eyes open and focus on a fixed point in the room.

- Now breathe in through your nose, slowly and steadily for a count of four;

- hold your breath for two counts;

- again, breathe out slowly and steadily through your nose for a count of four;

- and hold your breath for two counts.

- Repeat this for a few minutes or until you feel calm and relaxed.

Diaphragmatic breathing

Another way to use the respiratory system to limit anxiety and also improve overall health is to retrain yourself to breathe deeply from your diaphragm. The diaphragm is a large muscle situated at the base of our lungs (Figure 5). Abdominal muscles help to control this dome-shaped structure and give the lungs power to fully inhale and exhale, which is why many athletes work on their 'core' muscles and not just areas used in their specific sports. Throughout life poor posture and habits may result in chest breathing that over time can weaken the diaphragm. Place a hand on your chest – does it rise when you breathe in? Does your tummy suck in when you inhale also? If so, you are probably not engaging your diaphragm properly and your breathing will not be as efficient as it could be. Take a moment to watch the way a baby or young child breathes – you'll see their bellies expand when they inhale as they haven't yet formed the habit of shallow chest breathing.

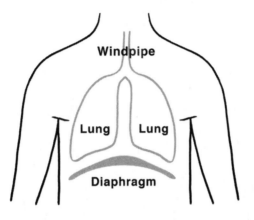

Figure 5 The diaphragm is a large dome-shaped muscle that plays a key part in respiration; it is located below the lungs as can be seen in this diagram

To improve your diaphragmatic breathing, try the exercise (Figure 6).

Diaphragmatic breathing exercise

- To do this technique, you first need to locate your diaphragm. Place one hand on your stomach with smallest finger directly above your belly button – your diaphragmatic muscles will be under your palm.

- Now position your other hand on your chest;

- inhale slowly and steadily through your nose and count to three;

- and exhale slowly and steadily for three counts whilst repeating the word 'relax' in your mind.

- You'll know if you're doing the exercise properly and breathing through your diaphragm if your bottom hand lifts outward as you breathe in and dips back when you exhale.

- While both inhaling and exhaling, try to relax the muscles in your shoulders and chest. Your top hand should feel still whilst breathing through your diaphragm – if it's not you're still breathing through your chest.

- Repeat five to 10 times or until you feel relaxed and calm is restored.

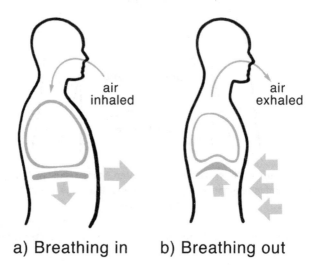

a) Breathing in   b) Breathing out

Figure 6 When breathing using your diaphragm, rather than your chest, your stomach will lift as you inhale and dip as you exhale

Mindfulness exercises

In Chapter 6 we discussed a type of therapy called mindfulness, which teaches people to live more in the moment in an effort to cope with general stress and/or the strain of having an unpredictable and intrusive illness like IBS. If you'd like to try a mindfulness approach but would prefer to do it yourself rather than attend a course, there is a vast range of books available on the topic. There are also smartphone apps, podcasts and online resources that you can explore if you'd like to delve more into this method. Here are some simple exercises that you can try to get a sense of what mindfulness techniques are like.

Fully immerse yourself in the mundane

You might wonder why you'd want to immerse yourself in mundane tasks – as previously mentioned, the core concept of mindfulness is to root ourselves in the present rather than being stuck in the past or preoccupied with things yet to happen in the future. By taking note of everyday movements and sensations we might just find contentedness in daily tasks, such as vacuuming the bedrooms, doing the washing up and even cleaning the oven.

Most of the time we are thinking about the long list of other chores we need to do, worrying about our kids or focusing on what we should have said in an argument yesterday rather than noticing each component of a task. Therefore, to begin immersing yourself mindfully in an everyday job, choose something you do on a regular basis; as an example, let's take doing the washing up as our exercise:

- Remember with all mindfulness techniques that it is natural for our thoughts to wander. If this happens, take note of the thought but try not to judge it or critically evaluate it; for instance, 'My diarrhoea was really bad this morning' can be categorised simply as a thought, nothing more, nothing less and then gently set adrift again.

- Notice the temperature and feel of the water as it flows from the tap.

- When adding the soap to the running water, observe the pattern of the bubbles, place your hands in the bubbles and feel the sensation.

- Feel the weight of each plate and cup before adding them to the sink. If your mind starts to meander and recalls what happened at dinner last night, take note of the thought but softly prod it away and focus again on placing the dish in the soapy water.

- Focus on the muscles and tendons you're using while washing the dishes. You may not have noticed this before even though you've probably washed the dishes many times in your life.

- Rather than trying to rush the task, savour each moment and movement. This may be a mundane job but by concentrating on the tiny details, you can create a sense of peace and tranquillity in your own home at the same time as doing chores.

See something for the first time

Find a natural object, perhaps a flower or plant, or even a natural surface like wood. If you're thinking that you've seen this flower/plant/surface countless times, then that's true; but it's also true that you may not have observed it mindfully before and this is the exercise. It's all too easy to skim over the beauty and serenity of the natural world when we're in pain and discomfort, and although this exercise won't necessarily rid you of your symptoms, it can help to reduce the heightened stress response that may be activated when we're dealing with a complex illness like IBS.

- After you've chosen your object, look at it for one or two minutes. Pick something from your close surroundings; there's no need to go out and buy something for this exercise as all the techniques in this chapter are things you can do immediately from home. If you can't find an object you like the look of, go outside and gaze at the clouds, or moon if it's night-time.

- As always, if thoughts glide into your mind (perhaps, 'Why am I doing this, it's so stupid!') acknowledge the thought and nudge it back into the ether.

- Now observe the object – really observe it as if you're an alien from another planet and it is the first time you've seen it.

- Notice the pattern of the grain on the wood or the dips and crater shadows of the moon. Explore the object; once you think you've identified every detail, look again – there is most probably something you missed at the beginning of the exercise.

- By grounding ourselves in the natural world it's possible to live in the moment and let our preoccupations and stresses melt away, even if only for a few seconds at first.

Slow down the pace

- While life may need to be lived at a breakneck pace in some circumstances, this mindfulness exercise helps to slow down our internal pace, which, in turn, will help us to not feel as if we're always a step behind. This may seem counter-intuitive but try it and see how you feel.

- Find an action that you carry out many times a day – for instance, sitting down. The action you choose needn't be physical in nature; it could be sensory, such as when you smell food, or a completely internal event, such as a type of thought (i.e. a self-critical thought).

- Every time you sit down, take a moment to shine a spotlight (metaphorically of course) on exactly where you are, what you're in the process of doing (e.g. about to start work/ watch TV/ eat dinner) and how you feel.

- Tune into your body and feel the sensation of the chair beneath you and your feet on the floor.

- Observe the moment.

- If you're using thoughts as your prompt, take note of where you are, what you're doing and how you feel, as if you're using a physical cue but here use the mindfulness technique to release the critical thought and let it float away into the atmosphere.

- Choose a prompt that you feel comfortable with. The purpose of the physical/sensory/cognitive reminder is to nudge you into the mindful practice numerous times a day.

By doing this on a daily basis, and with practice, you will find you can use mindfulness techniques at times of heightened stress. You can also combine the breathing techniques above with these mindfulness exercises into a personalised relaxation programme.

Dealing with panic attacks

Sometimes even when you've used the cognitive, breathing and mindfulness strategies outlined above to deal with anxiety, a situation can be overwhelming and result in a panic attack. The 'attack' itself can be terrifying, producing symptoms such heart palpitations/chest pain, shortness of breath, dizziness and, in some severe cases, a choking sensation. These symptoms can make people think they're having a heart attack but any cardiac sensations are short-lived and do not damage the heart.

Another common feature of panic attacks is hyperventilation, or 'over-breathing'. The tricky aspect of this is that hyperventilating can make the attack worse because you feel as if you can't inhale enough air. In reality, the opposite is true and you have too much oxygen when hyperventilating. Recalling from the earlier section on breathing techniques, this situation results in a lack of carbon dioxide, which in itself creates a number of symptoms – one of which, annoyingly, is shortness of breath. Hence, panic attacks and hyperventilation feed into one another so the key to dealing with a panic attack is to regulate breathing patterns in the first instance. Here are a few techniques to help with this:

- Paper bag method: You may have seen this in films or on TV and maybe even have thought it was nonsense. The difficulty with this method is having access to a paper bag; so if you find it works for you, you might want to consider adding a small paper bag to your emergency pack (below). Open the bag and place it on your face covering both your mouth and nose. Inhaling and exhaling into the bag will cause you to breath back in the carbon dioxide you've expelled, rather than taking in more oxygen. This will help to remedy the respiratory alkalosis (low carbon dioxide levels) and, in turn, the unpleasant sensations associated with a panic attack.

- Holding your breath: Of course you may not want to use a paper bag in public, which is completely understandable. So instead, simply hold your breath for as long as is comfortable for you. Like the paper bag method, this will reduce the amount of carbon dioxide you breathe out. If you can hold your breath for around 10–15 seconds, then repeat three or four times, the hyperventilation should diminish and you'll start to feel calmer.

Do use the cognitive and mindfulness techniques mentioned in this chapter on a regular basis as this will help to prevent over-breathing. Regular exercise (see Chapter 4) can also ameliorate the tendency to hyperventilate, as can retraining yourself to breathe using your diaphragm.

Take strength in others – support groups

'A massive thing that has improved my confidence is talking to other sufferers. One of my closest friends also suffers with GI problems and having someone to talk to openly and frankly about the embarrassing symptoms and how it makes you feel has been a godsend. Realising that you aren't alone is a big step towards "getting over it" in your head.'

Emily

As we saw in Chapter 2, social support is beneficial not just because we feel understood and legitimised; it also releases chemicals in our bodies that combat stress. There are numerous online support groups where you can post questions, collect information and feel part of a group that understands what you're going through. One research study actually looked at what people gained from these sorts of groups and in an analysis of 572 posted messages found emotional support, esteem-boosting, information sharing, networking, and practical assistance were provided by group members[48]. With regard to the informational support that was offered, this tended to be in the areas of symptom interpretation, illness management and interaction with healthcare professionals.

A slight word of warning though – please bear in mind that the information shared with online groups might not come from a reliable source so do double-check any suggestions before trying them. Also, it's better to join a moderated group (where someone, usually a volunteer, looks at messages that are submitted to make sure that only appropriate posts are published) as sometimes people can become more argumentative online than they would be in person.

Other self-help suggestions

'I make provision for a possible IBS attack, rather than letting that risk affect decisions about where I go and what I do. I have now settled into a pattern. I can predict my attacks and I know how to deal with each one so it has the minimum impact on my life.'

Emily

Emergency pack

If you feel very anxious about going out or travelling, it might be worth taking an 'emergency pack' with you when you leave the house. Primarily this is a comfort blanket as severe incidents are rare. However, just having the pack with you will often reduce the anxiety associated with going out, therefore making an acute diarrhoea episode even more improbable. Items you may want to include in your pack are, for example:

- medications such as Buscopan for stomach cramping

- diarrhoea relief tablets if you find these effective

- flushable wet wipes

- a change of underwear and sealable plastic bag (for soiled underwear – these can be rinsed and then put into the plastic bag to wash later at home)

- note cards with reminders of breathing exercises to calm you down if the anxiety starts to rise

- relaxation apps on your smartphone – these can also help, as can calming music.

Taking this pack with you shouldn't feel embarrassing or shameful. Many women carry a similar collection of items during menstruation (e.g. painkillers, sanitary pads, wipes, etc) so it is nothing to be ashamed of. Men commonly now also carry bags to hold all their personal items in, so a discrete washbag can be tucked away underneath magazines and other daily paraphernalia. But, as previously mentioned, simply taking these items can reduce the stress of a journey or outing and in turn the possibility of a flare-up.

Radar key

The charity Disability Rights UK has developed a National Key Scheme (NKS) that allows disabled people and those with health conditions to access locked public toilets throughout the UK, for instance in bus and train stations, shopping malls, cafés, pubs, etc (https://crm.disabilityrightsuk.org/radar-nks-key). By using this in conjunction with a toilet-finder app (there are many free apps of this kind available), you will be able to quickly and freely access facilities when you are out and about. In fact, to put your mind at rest you may want to use the toilet-finder app before you set out for the day so you know exactly where they are. Finally, remember to keep your radar key in your IBS emergency pack.

Summary

In this chapter we have explored a number of ways you can tackle your IBS in addition to the medical, nutritional and psychological treatments outlined in earlier chapters. These are all positive steps on your path to managing your IBS and regaining control of your life.

Now that you have the tools to start regaining control of your health, we will discuss in the next two chapters how our knowledge of the causes of IBS has changed and some of the differences between the way that doctors and patients think about the condition. Some of this information is quite technical; however, we hope you find it interesting, even in the sense of how research has moved on in the past decade.

Chapter 8

The evolution of understanding IBS:

early explanatory models and doctor and patient perspectives

We all have different opinions about what makes us healthy and what can make us ill. The way we think about health and illness changes over time due to our experiences, what we're told about a particular condition or symptoms (by our parents, doctors, the media, in school, etc) and also what information emerges from scientific studies. Many decades ago people thought smoking was good for our health and doctors even suggested people smoke cigarettes to overcome numerous health complaints! Of course, we know now that this is not the case but it took some time for this view to change.

> 'It is a short shift, biomedically-speaking, from saying that the cause of a disorder or the pathological explanation for its symptoms is unknown to assuming that the problem is psychosomatic or all "in people's heads".
>
> *Wainwright, Russell and Yiannakou*[49]

As the quote above implies, it's only a short step from 'We can't find anything wrong' through to 'There is nothing wrong' to 'It's all in your head'. However, hopefully the only people who now think this are people who don't really know about IBS. Unfortunately you might come across some of those people, in which case, tell them of all the biological and physiological factors that can cause IBS! This is the first of two chapters that look at the ways patients, doctors and researchers think about the causes of IBS and why some people seem more prone to the condition than others. These 'explanatory models' are important as they can influence the types of treatments that are offered, how friends and family might behave towards someone with IBS, what research is carried out by scientists and also how society views the illness.

To start off with, we explore older models of IBS and healthcare practitioner perspectives, and then move on to the views of those with IBS. In Chapter 9 we look at the way recent research has changed the way scientists think about IBS, which over time will trickle down to healthcare and society as a whole.

Explanatory models of IBS

Explanatory models of IBS are how people explain the different features of IBS – the causes, likely duration of the illness and treatment. These models are used to explain IBS by both healthcare professionals and patients. Sometimes the explanatory models used by healthcare professionals and patients differ.

Let's look at a very simple (fictitious) model in Figure 7.

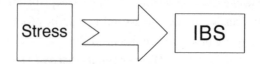

Figure 7 A simple model of IBS that only includes one possible reason for symptoms; here it is stress

The model shows that the researcher hypothesises that only one factor (stress) causes IBS. It isn't that helpful, because it doesn't tell us how the researcher believes stress causes or contributes to IBS.

The model could be:

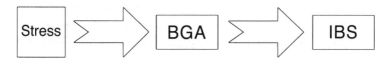

Figure 8 A more complex model of IBS that includes both stress and the brain–gut axis, illustrating that IBS is more complex than being simply due to stress

Figure 8 at least shows that stress leads to IBS via the brain–gut axis.

Non-fictitious models, unlike those above, are constructed from the latest scientific research. Models are constructed because the researchers believe their model can be useful for thinking about IBS. Other researchers will then look at the model, and carry out further research, which might lead to the addition or subtraction of other factors.

Staying with our fictitious example, other researchers might have found out that genetics play a part in IBS. Their research builds on the model so that it might now look like Figure 9.

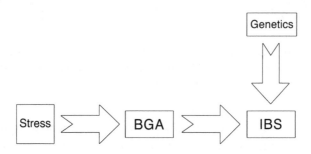

Figure 9 An even more complex model of IBS which includes stress, the brain–gut axis and also genetics to explain how IBS symptoms might occur

These models are not static; they change as more information becomes available.

Early models of IBS

As mentioned in Chapter 1, a commonly used model of IBS is the 'biopsychosocial model'. Researchers and healthcare professionals who accept this model believe that it's the one that can explain IBS better than others. The biopsychosocial model means that IBS is best explained by looking at the ways in which biological, psychological and social factors interact. Here is an example of a diagram of an early version of this model:

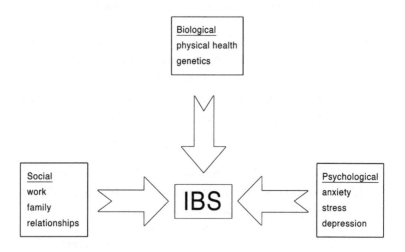

Figure 10 The 'biopsychosocial' model of IBS which includes biological, psychological and social factors that may play a part in the development of IBS symptoms

As IBS is a complex condition, the models are bound to be complex. As we have said before, simplistic ideas of IBS do not fit the picture of this illness.

Perspectives from healthcare professionals

Researcher Rachel Casiday and colleagues, from the Wolfson Research Institute at Durham University in the UK, wanted to understand general practitioners' (GPs') explanatory models for IBS[50]. They said that most doctors were aware that they didn't know what caused IBS and they felt frustrated because they couldn't really help their patients with their pain. Stress and tension were mentioned by every one of the 30 GPs. Many GPs felt that people with IBS didn't recognise the role stress played in IBS, although this is contrary to what we found. Many people we've spoken to have said that stress was a trigger. We must mention, though, that this article was written in 2009, so maybe things have changed? It was good to find, however, that GPs did mention that infection had a role in IBS.

In a more recent study, carried out in 2013, Elaine Harkness from Manchester University, together with other colleagues, conducted interviews with GPs in order to find out their views about IBS[51]. They focused on causes, diagnoses and treatments of IBS. It was very enlightening to find that all the GPs they spoke to thought that IBS was a real, accepted illness. The GPs believed that IBS was a complex condition and seemed to subscribe to the biopsychosocial model. Some of them even experienced IBS themselves. They recognised that IBS is sometimes difficult to deal with and mentioned the distressing effects of the condition. They mentioned giving advice to patients about lifestyle, diet and complementary treatments to manage IBS. They had fairly positive attitudes to people with IBS. Hopefully attitudes towards IBS and people with the illness are improving. However, none of the doctors was reported to have talked about the possibility of antibiotics or microbiota being involved in IBS (see Chapter 9), which was disappointing. Maybe in our next edition of this book, things will have changed further?

Patient perspective

In addition to uncovering doctors' views of IBS, Rachel Casiday and her colleagues carried out research with IBS patients[52]. Altogether, 51 people with a diagnosis of IBS were asked questions regarding their experience of IBS and their beliefs about the causes of the condition – in other words, the patients were asked to discuss their explanatory models. Most of them recalled a specific event that seemed to trigger the onset of IBS, such as pregnancy, some sort of illness or an accident that resulted in the need for strong pain medicine. Other patients didn't cite a particular triggering event but rather told the researcher that their symptoms were something to do with their individual make-up (which can perhaps be inferred as a genetic predisposition – more about this on page 131).

What was somewhat surprising to the researchers was that some of the patients didn't mention anything about the underlying cause of their IBS. Instead the interviewees talked more about issues that provoked flare-ups of symptoms, such as stress and certain foods. Therefore, it seems that explanatory models – thinking about the causes of IBS – were not as important to these patients as knowing what could aggravate the condition and therefore how it could be managed. This of course is not surprising if you have IBS!

'I was diagnosed when I was 17, by a consultant. He gave me tablets, but I can't remember what they were. I competed in athletics and had the best run of my life and just passed out on the last 100 metres; no reason; I can't remember a thing; it was awful. The doctor said it was possibly the medication and thus ended my athletics season early that year as teachers did not want to chance it, even if I stopped the medication. So from the word go I hated this diagnosis! It comes and goes; I think with stress or stressful situations it gets worse. Also, I read that anxiety is linked to the tummy, so I don't know if this has anything to do with it. My dad had severe anxiety and I think

I am a bit in denial that I have a little bit too as it is in these situations when things get worse.'

Maria

Explanatory models from research

So far we have looked at some fictitious models of IBS, some explanatory models that doctors hold, and we have also seen that some patients focus on symptoms and things that aggravate symptoms rather than models *per se*. As previously mentioned, explanatory models change all the time when new research is conducted – in fact, it is often the goal of researchers and scientists to try to fit all the pieces together and come up with new models. These models take some time to trickle down into healthcare as there needs to be a 'critical mass' of information for health bodies to update their models. (In the UK, this would be the National Institute for Health and Care Excellence (NICE) guidelines which healthcare practitioners use in the NHS.) In other words, many studies need to take place that have the same results so that on the balance of probabilities the model is the 'best fit' to the information at hand. There are numerous complex statistical ways of doing this, and also medical professionals and academics often meet to come to a consensus, such as when creating diagnostic criteria (see Chapter 1). This of course all takes time and, if you have IBS, you may not want to wait for this new understanding of your condition to trickle down to your GP. Many specialists pay attention to new research and often conduct it themselves so the models we are going to discuss in the next chapter will have been accepted and used by some medical professionals already. First, let's start by outlining the factors we now know are involved in IBS.

Factors involved in IBS

As we have said already many times in this book, IBS can be caused and maintained by many different factors. Different people may have a different set of factors acting together to produce symptoms – for example, your colleague may also have IBS but stress may not be a trigger for his symptoms. However, we are now seeing via high-quality research that there are some common mechanisms that underlie IBS. These are:

- Genetic predisposition

- Gastroenteritis: People who have had infectious gastroenteritis are more likely to suffer from IBS

- Use of antibiotics: These can cause a change in the number and type of gut bacteria, which disturbs the normal gut microbiota

- The BGA/HPA systems: Stress has adverse effects on these systems

- Inflammation of the gut mucosa: This suggests IBS is a low-grade inflammatory disease, which would lead to abdominal pain

- Increase in mast cells, which release chemicals that stimulate the enteric nervous system, causing altered motility of gut contents, pain and an increase in permeability in the gut (leakiness)

- Alterations in gut permeability: This would mean that certain substances that could trigger inflammatory responses could get through the intestinal wall

- Small intestinal bacterial overgrowth (SIBO): It might be the case that some people with IBS have an abnormally high number of 'bad' bacteria in the small bowel, which could lead to some of the symptoms of IBS

- Imbalance in gut microbiota – see Chapters 1 and 9

- Depression, anxiety, worry, sleep problems, psychiatric problems, etc mean that you are at greater risk for IBS than people without such problems. Such factors can have large effects on the BGA/ HPA systems, as mentioned in Chapter 1 and discussed in more detail in the next chapter.

Genetic predisposition

As we mentioned in Chapter 1, studies have consistently found that if your parents or grandparents had IBS, you stand a greater chance of having IBS than people in families with no history of the illness. Twin studies show that there is a higher percentage of identical twins having IBS than non-identical twins; this suggests that IBS is to some extent inheritable. For example, a large-scale study in Norway looked at 12,700 twins (both identical and non-identical) born between 1967 and 1979. In 1998, all the twins were sent a questionnaire asking them about any illnesses and symptoms including, 'Do you have, or have you ever had, irritable bowel syndrome?' Overall, 22.4% of the identical pairs had IBS, whereas only 9.1% of both non-identical twins reported having IBS[53]. This was seen by the researchers as statistically meaningful. Since identical twins share the same genetic code, but non-identical twins only share half of their genes with their twin (the same as any siblings) this research tells us that genetics plays a part in the development of IBS. Numerous other studies have found similar results but what these twin studies lack is an explanation of *how* genetics influences whether we experience IBS.

If IBS is in my genes, can I do anything about it?

As with all illnesses, if we know that we have a genetic predisposition to a condition it may seem that we have no control over our bodies. This, however, is not true; there are many things we *can* do to relieve the symptoms of IBS and take back control of our lives. Also, having a predisposition is just that, a tendency or susceptibility, rather than a life sentence, so if you have IBS and are worried that you may have passed it on to your children, please know that it's just not that simple. You may have heard of the 'nature or nurture' debate – are we born with certain problems or do illnesses (or behaviours) come about through things that happen to us throughout our lives? Yet again, the answer is not as straightforward as once thought. Our genetic code (or DNA sequence) and also DNA modifications interact with environmental factors. The study of the interactions between DNA and environmental factors is called 'epigenetics' and it is an exciting new scientific frontier.

Researchers have found that different genes (to date, over 60 different genes have been studied with regard to IBS) that control our individual characteristics, such as gender, neurobiology, personality and immunity, may interact with environmental factors like diet, infection, stress and trauma[54]. We will be looking at these characteristics and factors in more detail in the next chapter. What's important as a 'take home' message here is that there are many combinations of individual genetic and environmental risk factors (things that might make it more likely that you will develop IBS). These factors may result in changes in gastrointestinal motor and sensory function, or the brain–gut axis (BGA), with the end point being IBS symptoms. So the reasons why you became ill will not necessarily be the same reasons why someone you might know with IBS is unwell. In turn, different treatment strategies often work for different people, which is why we've discussed so many in this book.

Summary

In this chapter we have discussed a number of explanatory models of IBS and also outlined the factors that may be involved in the development of the disorder. The genetic predisposition to IBS was briefly explored and we have begun to think about models of IBS in terms of a number of factors interacting with one another. However, we haven't started to think about how these factors may lead to the mechanisms that underlie IBS, such as inflammation, gut permeability and changes in the gut microbiota.

In the next chapter we look more closely at the mechanisms and start to build up more sophisticated explanatory models of IBS based on recent research findings.

Chapter 9

Current models and new research into IBS

'It has recently become evident that microbiota, especially microbiota within the gut, can greatly influence all aspects of physiology, including gut–brain communication, brain function and even behaviour. Indeed, the initiation of large-scale metagenomic projects, such as the Human Microbiome Project, has allowed the role of the microbiota in health and disease to take centre stage.'

Cryan & Dinan[11]

We introduced you to gut microbiota in Chapter 1, where we discussed the trillions of micro-organisms that have evolved to live alongside us, primarily in our gut. Microbiota live on the inner surfaces of our intestines. There are many kinds of micro-organisms that live together harmoniously. The microbiota have a symbiotic relationship with us – that is, they get the benefit of a good environment with lots of nutrients, and we get benefits from the microbiota as their diversity contributes to normal gut function, and ensures nutrients are absorbed. They also play a part in the immune system. For instance, the gut microbiota develop a tolerance to toxins that normally lead to an immune response in our bodies. This means that, over time, we become immune to these toxins so that they do not produce an inflammatory response. However, the gut microbiota can be disturbed, leading to diseases such as IBD and IBS.

What can disturb the gut microbiota?

Infection and bacteria

'In 1998 I had a period of severe food poisoning that lasted six months. It was *Campylobacter* (my dad undercooked some chicken at a family BBQ). I was really ill. I shat myself (literally, not, sadly, metaphorically) in a job interview, passed out on a pedalo and missed out on most of the fun of being a fresher at uni by being constantly too ill to go out or do anything. Looking back, I've never been the same since that bout of food poisoning. I'm not sure if *Campylobacter* can cause permanent IBS symptoms and no doctor has been able to give me a clear answer. But now, in my head at least, that was the start of it.'

Justin

Justin's assertion that his bout of food poisoning led to his IBS may not be all that far off the mark. In general, campylobacter enteritis lasts for around seven days. However, research has shown that approximately 25% of people who have had this infection still experience symptoms six months later and between seven and nine per cent of those go on to develop IBS[55]. It seems that the length and severity of the initial infection can also have an impact on the likelihood of having IBS later on; there is a greater chance of developing IBS if the acute bout of campylobacter enteritis lasts for more than 21 days[56].

Further research has shown the link between gastroenteritis and IBS. In a large study based in Walkerton, Ontario, where there was a microbial contamination of the municipal water supply, researchers Vermeire and colleagues reported that in May 2000, over 23,000 residents developed acute gastroenteritis. Later it was found that over 32% of people developed IBS[57]. Other infections, such as with Salmonella bacteria, have been shown to be a risk for IBS[58]. Overall, studies have found that having acute gastroenteritis is a very strong risk factor for IBS. This risk increases with increased use of antibiotics and if you are depressed, stressed or anxious.

Some studies have found that people with IBS have a different profile of gut microbiota than people without. For instance, a reduction in the number of particular bacteria, such as lactobacilli and bifidobacteria, has been found in IBS patients[59]. These two types of bacteria are good for us, in that they have anti-inflammatory effects. In addition, people with IBS and IBD have increases in gut bacteria such as *E.coli* and *Salmonella*.

Small intestinal bacterial overgrowth (SIBO)

Some studies report that IBS patients are more likely to have an abnormally high number of bacteria in the small bowel. This can lead to abdominal pain, diarrhoea and bloating. (The small bowel is where most digestion takes place and should not contain bacteria; these should be in the large bowel where they ferment food that cannot be digested and absorbed in the small bowel.) However, the studies that looked at prevalence of SIBO were not consistent, one finding 80% of people with IBS having SIBO, and others finding only 10%. So at the moment we don't know whether SIBO is important in IBS.

Antibiotics

A groups of researchers carried out a review of the short- and long-term effects of antibiotics on the microbiota[60]. They showed that antibiotics alter the gut microbiota, disturbing the balance in the gut, although several weeks after stopping the drugs the microbiota had recovered. So a short course of antibiotics when needed is obviously not too bad as these drugs are necessary for some acute infections. However, studies that focused on the long-term effects of taking antibiotics show that the microbiota don't get back to normal until 12 weeks after stopping the drugs.

What helps the microbiota?

It has been found that pre- and probiotics (see Chapter 5) are better for helping with IBS symptoms than placebo, or dummy, pre- and probiotics (capsules made to look like the real thing but not containing any active substance). However, like other drugs and treatments, they won't work for everyone – but unlike drugs, they don't have any damaging side effects. For instance, studies have shown that consuming high-cocoa drinks instead of low-cocoa drinks is better for your microbiota (Chapter 5). High-cocoa chocolate will also work: after consuming high levels of cocoa, the good bacteria bifidobacteria and lactobacilli show a significant increase, and also the bad bacteria clostridia a significant decrease.

Gut motility

Microbiota have an effect on gut motility (how fast or slowly the contents of the gut move through the bowels). However, the opposite is also true – if your gut motility changes there will be effects on your microbiota[61]. Changes here mean you have noticed that your bowel habits have altered from constipation to diarrhoea (speeded up) or from diarrhoea to constipation (slowed down), or you might have alternation of constipation and diarrhoea.

Does stress, or trauma, play a part in IBS?

'I am stone-cold convinced that my IBS is related to stress and emotional upset. Each flare-up that I have occurs during stressful times for me; worry, overwork, etc. Despite keeping a food diary, I still have not been able to fully pinpoint a dietary cause though, but what I know for certain is that my emotional state is the major cause. I also suffer from depression and anxiety and panic disorder, so this impacts on my IBS.'

Nancy

Early life trauma

Many studies have found that severe stress in early life seems to play a part in the later development of IBS. A very interesting study carried out by researchers in the Netherlands looked at whether babies who were born around the time of the Second World War were more likely to have the symptoms of IBS as adults. During this time in the Netherlands there was a terrible famine due to the retreating Nazis destroying all food and also the means to grow food, hence many people would have lived in near-starvation circumstances. Tamira Klooker and colleagues studied the life history of 816 men and women with IBS and found that those who had experienced the horrors of war at a very early age were indeed more likely to have IBS[62]. Furthermore, the longer the children were within these severe wartime conditions, the more likely they were to develop IBS. But it should be noted that within this particular study it is not possible to say that severe stress caused IBS as the children may also have been undernourished and infectious illness would have been rife.

Sexual and emotional abuse in early life

Even though the wartime study could not tell us for certain whether early life trauma leads to IBS, there have been many studies that have found that people who have been sexually or emotionally abused at a young age have an increased risk of having a chronic illness later in life. IBD and IBS have been particularly associated with these factors. Research carried out in the 1990s consistently demonstrated a correlation between abuse and IBS. As with the wartime study, it's important for us to appreciate the difference between a *correlational* study and one that can be used to determine *causation*. Correlational research merely tells us that there appears to be a link between two variables – that is, something that can be measured and is of interest to us, in this case abuse and IBS. But there may be other factors at play that are actually more important than the variables we are looking at, but of course we wouldn't know this at the time. Again, this is why explanatory models change – new scientists and researchers may wonder if different variables are in fact more important to the development of an illness and then test these. This would still be correlational research but other scientists may conduct experimental work that can tell us about causation and the mechanisms that may lead one variable to be linked to another. We will look at studies that have investigated these mechanisms later in this chapter, but first let's consider if the relationship between early life abuse and IBS is as definitive as once thought.

Big 'T' or little 't' trauma

We are now realising that trauma can come in many different forms. For someone to be affected by trauma there doesn't neces-sarily have to be a major event, such as the abuse mentioned above, death of a loved one or witnessing violence (e.g. wartime conflict). These are known as Big 'T' traumas. People can also experience little 't' traumas, such as growing up in a household that lacked love and security, bullying and victimisation, continual failures in life, and minor accidents. Little 't' trauma differs from Big 'T' trauma as it is the gradual build-up of daily hurts that may lead to health problems. In other words, a short bout of bullying may not affect us (and will affect different people to different degrees) but constant, unrelenting victimisation where we can't see a way out becomes a trauma to us and can lead to many different types of illness.

Evidence for little 't' trauma in IBS

A group of researchers at the School of Medicine and Biomedical Sciences within the University at Buffalo in New York State questioned whether family life and the way people were treated on an everyday basis (little 't' trauma) were more important considerations when thinking about IBS than acute childhood abuse (Big 'T' trauma). The researchers collected information from 81 people on both types of trauma; in this study parenting style was used as a measure of little't' trauma. The parenting style questions looked at whether the people with IBS had parents who were emotionally warm or cold towards them during childhood, if the household had an atmosphere of hostility and/or rejection, whether there was neglect at home, and also if 'undifferentiated rejection' was experienced (i.e. withdrawal of affection that was not clearly aggressive or neglectful *per se*). Somewhat surprisingly, the results showed that these negative parenting styles were related to IBS symptoms, but acute abuse was not[63]. This is surprising because one might expect both types of trauma, both Big 'T' and little 't', to be linked to IBS but not just one. Hence, little 't' trauma may be just as important, if not more so, when thinking about IBS than Big 'T' trauma.

Trauma and hypersensitivity

It is thought that traumatic stress, such as sexual abuse in the early years, has long-lasting effects on the brain–gut axis/hypothalamus–pituitary–adrenal axis (BGA/HPA) systems (page 13). The gut might be sensitised to stress so that any later acute and/or continuing stress may trigger an abnormal response in the BGA/HPA systems. It's a bit like being sensitive to noise. People who are exposed to loud music may become extra-sensitive to noise. People with migraine, ME/CFS and other disorders often become much more aware of sound and any later exposure to noise will have a much larger effect on them than on other people. Another example would be someone who has had a bad experience – for instance, being attacked. She or he would naturally be much more aware than other people of the sound of footsteps approaching, as discussed in Chapter 1 (page 13).

Traumatic effects in early life seem to sensitise the gut so that later stress has a bigger effect on abused people, amplifying their experience of IBS in comparison with people who did not experience traumatic events. Other 'stresses' which may have the same effects are post-traumatic stress, anxiety and worry, and chronic stress due to work or relationship problems. For instance, marital conflict has been shown to affect the HPA axis and compromise the immune system, which may cause symptoms to worsen.

Integrated model of IBS

In Chapter 1 we mentioned that the Big Brain (CNS – the central nervous system) communicates with the Little Brain (ENS – the gut, or 'enteric' nervous system). This interaction is called the brain–gut axis (BGA). Communications are two-way, from the CNS to the ENS and from the ENS to the CNS. The BGA ensures that everything relating to the GI system is in balance. Changes in the CNS or gut may disturb the intestinal microbiota. On the other hand, changes in the microbiota, such as by infection or antibiotics, will have effects on the Big Brain. Stress which affects the Big Brain can also lead to changes in your microbiota, and vice versa.

Based on research in 2009, researchers Collins and Bercik constructed a model (figure 11) that they think applies to the ways in which IBS can develop[64]. They knew that gastroenteritis, antibiotic use and stress (labelled infection, antibiotics or other factors) produce changes to the microbiota. (On the model this is labelled perturbation of the microbiota; 'perturbation' just means a change, in the microbiota in this case). They found that these changes lead to low-grade inflammation and the inflammation leads to gut dysfunction, which leads to symptoms of IBS (symptom generation). They also showed that changes to the microbiota (perturbation) have influences on the brain, which lead to altered behaviour, perhaps anxiety or worry. They labelled this 'psychiatric co-morbidity' which is just another name for psychological problems that people often have when they develop a chronic illness or disease. It doesn't mean you have a psychiatric illness.

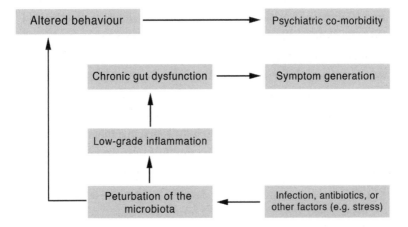

Figure 11 Researchers Collins and Bercik's (2009) integrated model of IBS which shows how the intestinal microbiota may be involved

Note that in order to read this diagram correctly, you need to read it from the bottom up starting from the bottom right-hand box, 'Infection, antibiotics, or other factors (e.g. stress)'.

Our updated IBS model

'I tend not to talk about "IBS" as the problem is altered tolerance, gut permeability and disordered peristalsis arising from a disruption in the GI immune and neuroendocrine system.'

Dr Amolak Bansal, Consultant Immunologist

Although we believe that the Collins and Bercik model is much more comprehensive than earlier models of IBS, we think that there are additional factors that can be included which have come out of research studies. These may heighten our understanding of the condition and the way that treatment can be developed.

Gut permeability

The gut mucosa houses the largest mass of immune cells in our body (Chapter 1). Although this barrier is usually very effective and protects us from illness, we do know that mild irritants, toxins and pathogens can actually open the junctions made by epithelial cells and increase gut permeability. The role of permeability in the gut is not completely known. However, there is evidence of abnormal permeability in IBS patients, particularly those with IBS-D[65]. Increased gut permeability has been indicated in a range of illnesses, including diabetes, Crohn's disease, multiple sclerosis and numerous autoimmune conditions. Hence, this issue might also be important in IBS.

Trauma and the gut mucosa

Research in animals (rats in this instance) has shown that trauma in early life and chronic stress can indeed lead to changes in the gut mucosa. These changes can affect gut permeability by allowing larger molecules to move across the barrier than would normally be expected in a healthy gut[66, 67]. These studies also showed that 'mast cells' were affected by stress and trauma.

Mast cells

'Mast cells' are immune cells involved in protecting us against pathogens and they also help regulate intestinal permeability. One study showed not only that there was an increased number of mast cells in the lining of the gut mucosa of people with IBS compared with healthy people, but also that the closer the mast cells were to the colonic nerve endings, the more intense and more frequent was the pain or discomfort[68]. This would naturally lead to abdominal pain and can also lead to an increase in permeability of the gut.

Immune activation

Research looking at results from biopsies following a colonoscopy (see Chapter 3, page 45) has also found that more people with IBS have immune activation than people without IBS. Half the 77 IBS patients in this study could be diagnosed with colitis based on the inflammation found in the biopsies. But even in those patients that had 'normal' results that were within the medical ranges to exclude the diagnosis of other disorders like IBD, there were clear indications of immune activation in the biopsies[69].

Disordered peristalsis

In a study that looked at IBS and ulcerative colitis, researchers found that there were changes in important neurotransmitters in those with both conditions[70]. The outer layer of the gut mucosa is formed of smooth muscle tissue, which contracts and relaxes to help us digest our food. This movement has the technical name 'peristalsis' and is controlled in part by neurotransmitters, specifically serotonin. (We looked at serotonin earlier on page 57.) So if there is an alteration in our neurotransmitters, this can lead to changes in peristalsis (disordered peristalsis) which will then affect gut motility. Indeed, the researchers found that there were numerous signs of disruption in the signalling function of serotonin in those with IBS and ulcerative colitis.

Arroll and Dancey model of IBS

In order to make sense of all this dense information, we've constructed the model of IBS shown below in Figure 12. Here we see that there are a number of triggers that may kick-start the illness and there will undoubtedly be a genetic contribution to whether these acute factors then develop into IBS. What we're interested in presenting here are the changes, or 'mechanisms', that have been found in IBS and that can explain why you experience some of the distressing symptoms associated with it. But we also want to include strategies that you can use to diminish your symptoms and help to rectify some of the physiological disturbances found in IBS. We believe that BGA and HPA (see page 13) play an important part in IBS, both in its commencement and resolution.

So, let's look at Figure 12 – if you start at the top, you'll see the 'genetic predisposition' banner as not everyone who experiences IBS triggers will necessarily develop the condition (see Chapter 8). Next we have the 'triggers and symptom aggravators'; we included both triggers and aggravators because IBS can be a fluctuating illness, where people can improve but if something happens, like a stressful event or needing to take antibiotics, symptoms can happen again even if they had stopped for a while.

Moving down the model, we have a section called 'mechanisms'. This section of the model has two sides – let's focus on the right-hand side for now. We've added negative changes to the microbiota, increased gut permeability, increased immune activation and disordered peristalsis, but this is not to say that there aren't more mechanisms at play in IBS – these are simply the ones we view as important at the present time. These mechanisms can give rise to IBS symptoms.

After symptoms have been ongoing people usually seek out help, so next we've added a box called 'treatments and self-help'. These strategies should lead to improvements in symptoms; but of course if symptoms are decreasing it means that something is going on with the underlying mechanisms, such as they're being resolved. Hence the box that includes positive changes in the microbiota, decreases in gut permeability, lowered immune activation and normalised peristalsis has an arrow that leads to 'symptom reduction'. Importantly, it is the BGA/HPA pathway that links treatments and self-help to the beneficial changes in the IBS mechanisms.

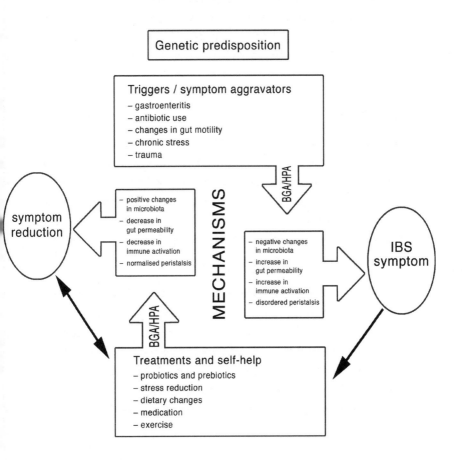

Figure 12 The Arroll and Dancey model of IBS – Our model of the condition which includes the interaction between possible mechanisms involved in IBS, triggers and ways to reduce symptoms.

It must be noted, however, that symptom reduction and improvements in IBS are not static end points – IBS is a chronic condition so the interventions you use may need to be ongoing and care taken to manage any flare-ups, hence the two-way arrow between 'symptom reduction' and the treatments and self-help box on the model.

But even though IBS is a long-term condition, we hope that the information in this book will help you find your best way to deal with its symptoms, whether this is a mixture of medicines and self-help, psychological treatment and moderate exercise or stress reduction and support from friends and relatives (for example).

Summary

In this chapter we have reviewed some of the newer and emerging research that has given us more clues to the underlying nature of this complex condition. The picture is not yet complete and even when, or if, we do have greater understanding of IBS the treatments may remain the same for some time. But nevertheless we hope that the information here has shown you the exciting new insights that researchers are uncovering about the condition.

The next and final chapter is directed at family, friends and colleagues. You may want to discuss the topics in this chapter with them or simply hand them this book to read for themselves. Gaining support from those around you will help to reduce the isolation that can come from having an invisible illness like IBS. So once you've read the next chapter, do consider opening up an avenue of conversation on the subject as this will help those close to you to help you.

Chapter 10

Guide for family, friends and colleagues

Note to readers with IBS

This chapter is for the family, friends, colleagues and other members of your support group. For simplicity's sake here we will just call them your 'friend'. Sometimes it can be difficult to ask for the help we need so you may want to give this chapter to a friend or family member as a basis for starting a conversation about your IBS. But you may not want to talk about your condition directly, so you could give the person concerned this chapter and just say it's for him/her to think about. Either way, the ideas below are aimed directly at others who can help you when your symptoms are at their worst and also help you get the best out of life.

For family, friends and colleagues

It is not always easy to understand what a person is going through when they have an illness. People understand what it's like to have a cold, a headache or flu, but unless they have experienced IBS – or cancer, for that matter, or any other illness – then it is hard to really understand what's going on. If you are in the position of having to live with or care for someone with an illness, then the illness will affect you as well. Research has shown that families of people with illness share a significant weight or burden. They may have to take over some of the responsibilities of the person who is ill. There has been a lot of research showing how the life-threatening illness of a loved one who, say, has cancer, negatively affects families or care-givers. Studies have shown that partners of patients with IBS also carry a significant burden, compared with people who have healthy partners. The more severe the IBS, the greater the burden is on the partner. So ensure that you treat yourself gently as well.

Although IBS is invisible, it is a very real illness

There are many conditions where people look fine, even very well, but they are in fact in a great deal of discomfort and pain. Other 'invisible illnesses' include IBD, fibromyalgia, migraine, ME/CFS, balance disorders such as Meniere's disease, rheumatoid arthritis, epilepsy … the list goes on and on. It can be hard to have symptoms yet look fine from the outside.

Everyone has experienced some sort of pain or discomfort at some time. Try to remember when you last had a headache or other bodily pain. You probably looked perfectly alright to everyone else but you may have been feeling unwell on the inside. Now imagine feeling like this constantly.

People with IBS are subjected to a double whammy. Not only do they feel rotten, but there is often a lack of support from those close to them, such as family members and friends. Work and recreational situations can also be challenging as without outward signs of ill-health, someone with a condition like IBS can feel very isolated indeed. People with the condition often find it very hard to acknowledge their IBS and in turn to discuss it with others due to the embarrassing nature of the symptoms.

In addition to this, IBS can also attract stigma as it is a complex condition that does not have a single cause or test that can pinpoint a disease process – that is, there are no scans, investigations or blood tests which can show that a person has IBS. This does not mean that IBS is not 'real'; rather that it's a multifaceted condition and we are only just learning about the physiological processes underlying it. For example, factors such as the use of antibiotics, gastrointestinal infections and life experiences appear to interact with a person's genes to produce the symptom of IBS.

So, someone with IBS may appear perfectly fine – in fact, almost anyone will say 'good' or 'well' if you ask them how they are. This does not mean that IBS is not a debilitating and intrusive illness. All it means is that your friend, brother or workmate who has IBS is trying to put his or her best face on.

What you can do to help...

Simply acknowledge your friend's experiences as real and distressing. You don't need to know everything about IBS or understand all the complex theories behind it; just by accepting what your friend says about how he or she is feeling is a great help and support.

IBS can take a long time to be diagnosed ... and is often misdiagnosed

Your friend may have to consult various different doctors and have a number of tests before a diagnosis of IBS is obtained. Conversely, a GP may have diagnosed IBS very quickly but your friend may still feel that something else is the cause of his/her symptoms. You may feel like this journey is anything but straightforward and you would be correct. IBS does not have an easy test to confirm diagnosis so even if someone has this diagnosis, it could turn out later that they really have a different disease. Both the struggle for an initial diagnosis and the feeling of frustration engendered by being misdiagnosed can be difficult for the person with IBS symptoms, and this is on top of feeling unwell, of course.

As IBS is a complex illness and the road to diagnosis and treatment can be rather bumpy, it is good for those with this condition to develop a collaborative relationship with doctors and healthcare professionals. This can be a tricky relationship to build as people with invisible illnesses often feel ignored and not taken seriously by medical professionals.

What you can do to help...

Help your friend with his symptom diary if he wants you to. (He may not and this should be respected.) Those close to us can often see other signs and symptoms, such as fatigue or bad temper, which the person with IBS may not note explicitly. Including this information in a symptom log can help doctors to get an accurate picture of the illness as a whole and aid diagnosis and treatment. Also, if your friend is getting very frustrated with his/her GP, support him by listening to his concerns non-judgementally and giving reassurance that relief will be found even if it takes time and changes in lifestyle.

IBS can make a person very isolated

At first glance, you may not think that IBS is the type of illness that would lead to isolation. For instance, you may wonder why your colleague can't get out and about like she used to do (or, can't travel far/go out to a meal etc). However, some of the symptoms of IBS can come about incredibly suddenly. Just imagine that you're on a packed commuter train. This train may or may not have a toilet. The toilet may or may not be in working order. Even in a best-case scenario, it may be impossible to access the toilet due to the crowds. If you can access the services, you may feel extremely embarrassed about some of the unpleasant consequences of IBS symptoms, such as noise and smell. But the fear that you might not be able to get to the toilet, the toilet isn't working or there isn't a toilet on the train, could be enough to stop you from making the trip at all. You can probably imagine other, less severe situations that could feel frightening for a person who experiences a sudden onset of IBS symptoms.

Even in a less desperate situation, it may be uncomfortable for someone with IBS to engage in social activity. A huge proportion of our social interactions take place with an accompaniment of food and drink. Think about it for a moment – how many times do you meet with friends and work colleagues socially without eating or drinking something? In most cultures, there won't be many get-togethers that don't involve some type of food consumption. Eating (and to a lesser extent drinking) in public may have also become a terrifying prospect for a person with IBS if he is symptomatic. This can then lead to isolation as your workmate may continually turn down offers for dinner and after-work drinks.

What you can do to help...

Try to think of things to do that are still of interest to you and your friend, which don't necessarily involve lengthy commutes or meals out. For instance, if your friend used to enjoy going to a football match but now he seems reluctant, it may be that he's worried about being able to access a toilet easily. Instead, suggest that you both watch a game in his house or at a local pub. This way the worry about being near a toilet will be reduced and your friend can benefit from some very important social interaction (unless of course your team loses). If you used to go out for dinner all the time but now don't, see if he instead would like to pop round to watch a film. Of course both of these activities *might* involve food also, so you may want to broach the subject and ask if there's anything your friend would like or say it's fine for him to bring his own snacks.

The IBS person will be an expert in IBS!

Sometimes we as friends and family members can become overly protective and watchful of our loved ones when they are unwell. This can be counter-productive as continually asking someone if he is okay may lead to anxiety in that person. Stress and anxiety can actually worsen and/or trigger symptoms (see below). So, whilst we should be aware of the limitations that IBS may impose on some of the areas of a person's life, it's also helpful for your relationship with your friend, partner or workmate to keep in mind that he is the expert in his own health and illness.

Similarly, we want to help our friends recover so it can be very tempting to offer advice. This again can make someone with IBS, or any long-term condition, anxious as an underlying tone of 'you're not trying hard enough to get better' may be perceived, even if it is not intended. You may feel excited to have read in a magazine that a new diet plan has led to the complete cure of a person with IBS and you want to share this news. Please take a moment and consider that your friend is working with his doctors to find the best treatment plan for his individual set of symptoms. Not everyone with IBS is the same and so a therapy that has worked for one person may not work for the next.

What you can do to help...

Although it is important to make some changes to accommodate times when your friend may have IBS symptoms, it's also very important not to infantilise or treat him as if he is fragile. So treat your friend as you would normally, but with an awareness that alterations in activities and schedules may need to be made. Your friend probably thinks about IBS far too much already so although you shouldn't shy away from a conversation if he wants to talk about the illness, it needn't be the focus of all conversation.

IBS can be unpredictable

With regard to activities and social arrangements, another aspect of IBS that can make life a bit miserable is its unpredictable nature and symptom flare-ups. Even when someone has found a good way forward in terms of treatment, symptoms can occur without any apparent trigger. This means that some plans will be cancelled at the last minute. This can create a huge sense of guilt in the person with IBS. He may have been a very reliable person before developing IBS and now seems to cancel meeting up on a regular basis. Your friend is still the reliable person he always was; it is just that these symptom flare-ups are beyond his control. It's important not to take cancellations personally or feel offended by them. In fact, if your friend knows that you will totally understand if he has to cancel, the chances are that it won't happen. Yet again, this is to do with how stress affects the illness (see below).

Also, by being flexible with your friend this will allow him to avoid a lack of planning and/or over-scheduling, both of which can worsen IBS. Having a regular routine, with nice social time built in, is essential in managing the symptoms of IBS. People with unpredictable illnesses can often avoid making plans when they feel unwell and then to compensate they will arrange many outings when they feel a bit better to try to catch up. But of course this over-scheduling can then instigate a return of symptoms, resulting in cancellations that then need to be rebooked. This 'boom-and-bust' pattern is detrimental for people with chronic illness.

What you can do to help...

Make your friend aware that it is no problem at all if he needs to cancel or postpone arrangements, even at very short notice. Flexibility and understanding on your part can help your friend immensely while he sets a new routine. This will also allow him to feel more in control of his life in the face of a seemingly uncontrollable illness.

Even though stress may exacerbate IBS symptoms, IBS is not a psychological illness

Stress and anxiety will make any illness worse. Indeed, even a healthy person can feel very unwell physically when experiencing a great deal of stress – for example, he may feel his heart pounding, start sweating or even feel nauseous. These sensations during acute stress are normally short-lived and don't cause anyone health problems. But when someone is unwell already or if stress is chronic, the physiological changes that occur in our bodies during stressful times can make an illness worse. This is because stress can adversely impact on our body's immune system.

Have you ever noticed that you seem to come down with a cold, not during a very stressful time, but just when you have a moment to relax? For instance, have you ever seemed to pick up bugs on holiday or around Christmas time just when all the stress of getting work completed so you can actually have time off has subsided? This is because your body has been helping you deal with the pressures but in doing so your immune system may not be at its best to fight off infections. However, you wouldn't then think your cold or cough was due to stress in itself would you? You would still understand that you've contracted a virus or other type of infection.

Therefore, stress such as problems at work, relationship difficulties or more general pressures, such as feeling the need to conform to certain 'norms' (e.g. 'I must earn a lot of money to have worth') can have an impact on people with and without chronic conditions like IBS.

What you can do to help...

It can be hard for people to ask for support so give some thought to the stresses that your friend may have. Of course, simply experiencing IBS is stressful in itself but there are many ways that you may be able to help to reduce stress. These can be emotional, like acknowledging and accepting his illness experience as mentioned above. But support can also be more practical. Perhaps your friend has been finding his symptoms to be particularly bad first thing in the morning. Therefore, you may want to offer some help with the school run to take a bit of the pressure off him/her at the time when he is most symptomatic. Even if you can't do this every day, a small period of respite can often make a difference to a person with a chronic illness.

IBS can lead to depression

So far in this chapter, specifically for the family, friends, close acquaintances and work colleagues of those with IBS, we've highlighted that this condition is complex and the symptoms of IBS can lead to a person becoming quite isolated. Considering the misconceptions others may hold about IBS, the embarrassment and stigma that still surrounds toilet issues and the restrictions in activity that IBS symptoms can cause, it is easy to see how a person with IBS could start to feel down. Understanding that having an illness like IBS can make someone feel depressed is important for the way that you interact with them.

Also it's not just the limitations on daily life that can lead an individual with IBS to become depressed; immune activation can lead to feelings of low mood. People with IBS have often experienced infections or trauma which may instigate an immune response. When our immune system is set into action by an infection or injury, there are many consequences. We won't go into all of the physiology and biochemistry here, but small proteins called cytokines are released as an innate immune defence mechanism to protect our bodily systems when a threat is detected. However, the release of cytokines can have some unfortunate consequences such as fever, fatigue, loss of libido and also depression. Try and think about when you last had flu or a bad cold. Did you feel rather low? It may not have been the constantly runny nose and fever that were making your feel this way but rather your body's inflammatory response.

What you can do to help...

If your friend seems to be having a bad case of the blues, telling him/her to look on the bright side may not be the most useful way to approach the situation. Under these circumstances, the most important quality for you to possess as a friend is patience. It can be exceptionally difficult for us to see our friends feeling so low and we may tire of hearing about someone's health problems. However, please know that your friend is actively trying to help him/herself by researching his condition and attempting to find a treatment package that will help. Being prepared to hear the answer 'rubbish' to the common question of 'How are you?' may seem a trivial thing, but actually, staying the course with your friend when he is at his lowest without judgement is invaluable.

For partners and spouses – maintaining a sexual relationship when someone has IBS

Difficulty in maintaining a fulfilling sex life is a commonly reported consequence of IBS, noted in surveys and research by both men and women. Sex drive, or 'libido', can be affected, sex can become painful and also the embarrassing characteristics of IBS can turn a once active and satisfying sexual relationship into a frustrating and problematic area. These difficulties can result in a complete absence of sex in a partnership and this can impact on other areas of the relationship. So even though this can be a tricky subject to broach, it is necessary for both your and your partner's overall well-being.

The key here is open and honest communication. Of course this is easier said than done, so if you feel you and your partner need additional support on this issue, don't be embarrassed to ask your

GP or healthcare provider for guidance. You might be referred to a specialist counsellor who can guide the way to frank and non-judgemental communication. The counsellor may also be able to suggest other ways to create intimacy even when symptoms are present.

What you can do to help...

Although it may be difficult, try your best not to place blame onto your partner for a reduction in sexual activity. Having IBS is not his fault and you can both work back towards a good-quality sex life together. There are many ways to foster intimacy; for instance kisses and cuddles can act as a bond just as sexual acts can. Someone with IBS may not feel at all attractive, so reassure your partner that the IBS hasn't taken any desirability away from them. Most importantly, be honest and willing to find ways to share a sex life even if this means asking your GP for a referral to a specialist counsellor.

Summary

To recap, IBS is an unpredictable illness and can significantly disrupt a person's life. There are many factors involved in the development of IBS and stress is one such factor that you, as a friend, partner or close work colleague, can help to reduce. Also, by understanding the unpredictable nature of IBS, you'll be in a better position to support your friend and see that the changes in his behaviour are due to the illness, not the person. Therefore, in summary, the tips to helping are:

- Never question the existence of IBS, even if your friend looks and seems well

- Be patient with the process of diagnosis and finding an effective treatment – it can take time

- Try not to be over-protective or treat the person with IBS as if he is fragile

- Try to avoid giving advice, even if well-intentioned

- Be willing to find IBS-friendly activities that are still of interest to you both

- Understand that plans may be cancelled at short notice

- Offer practical support, such as help with the children, shopping, housework, gardening, etc

- If IBS is affecting your sexual relationship or damaging your relationship overall, seek external and professional support.

Overall, simply being there and accepting that the person with IBS is trying their best to overcome this debilitating and still misunderstood condition will be an invaluable support. IBS is an embarrassing and stigmatised illness that can challenge someone's very sense of self and belief in their body. Support, whether emotional or practical, can limit the likelihood of depression and isolation, factors which we know are detrimental to us all.

Overall summary and conclusions

People who have illnesses such as IBS have a great deal to cope with: from first experiencing confusing and embarrassing symptoms, to struggling to gain a diagnosis and then perhaps a lengthy journey to find effective treatments. In all of the invisible illnesses that we have studied over the years, we've found common threads. These are not necessarily to do with the symptoms themselves, but rather the impact on a person's life. By having an illness that no one can see, it can be difficult to gain the support and understanding that is needed to deal with it; not just the illness, but life in general. Chronic, non-life-threatening conditions, where the symptoms are experienced by most people at some point in their life (for instance with the occasional infection or virus) can also be trivialised by others: 'Oh yes, I get a dippy tummy too at times and isn't it awful, dear, but nothing to worry about really is it?' These factors can leave you feeling angry, hurt, frustrated and isolated, not knowing where to turn for general support or for specific advice to manage symptoms. Whilst we know that this book isn't a magic pill that can rid you of your IBS symptoms in one fell swoop, we hope that it has provided you with enough information to seek out the appropriate diagnosis and treatment, as well as some ideas on how you can integrate dietary changes, stress-reduction techniques and other hints and tips to limit the impact of this most distressing condition on your life.

We'd like to end with this message from a fellow person with IBS:

> 'Don't let IBS be something that stops you from living your life. Try to figure out what causes your IBS to flare up and work with it.'
>
> *Kwilole*

References

1. Khanbhai A, Sura DS. Irritable Bowel Syndrome for Primary Care Physicians. *British Journal of Medical Practitioners* 2013;6(1):a608.

2. Babic T. Sex Differences in GABAergic Neurotransmission to Gastric-Projecting DMV Neurons. *The FASEB Journal* 2015;29(1 Supplement):820-4.

3. Dancey CP, Backhouse S. Overcoming IBS: practical help in coping with Irritable Bowel Syndrome. Robinson; 1993.

4. Dancey CP, Backhouse S. IBS: A complete guide to relief from Irritable Bowel Syndrome: Robinson. 1997.

5. Dibonaventura MD, Prior M, Prieto P, Fortea J. Burden of constipation-predominant irritable bowel syndrome (IBS-C) in France, Italy, and the United Kingdom. *Clinical & Experimental Gastroenterology* 2012;5:203-12.

6. Card TR, Siffledeen J, Fleming KM. Are IBD patients more likely to have a prior diagnosis of irritable bowel syndrome? Report of a case-control study in the General Practice Research Database. *United European Gastroenterology Journal* 2014;2(6):505-12.

7. Arroll MA, Dancey CP. Invisible Illness: Coping with misunderstood conditions. Sheldon Press; 2014.

8. Stenner PH, Dancey CP, Watts S. The understanding of their illness amongst people with irritable bowel syndrome: a Q methodological study. *Social Science & Medicine* 2000;51(3):439-52.

9. Gladman LM, Gorard DA. General practitioner and hospital specialist attitudes to functional gastrointestinal disorders. *Alimentary Pharmacology & Therapeutics* 2003;17(5):651-4.

10. Drossman DA, Dumitrascu DL. Rome III: New standard for functional gastrointestinal disorders. *Journal of Gastrointestinal & Liver Disease* 2006;15(3):237-41.

11. Cryan JF, Dinan TG. Mind-altering microorganisms: the impact of the gut microbiota on brain and behaviour. *Nature Reviews Neuroscience* 2012;13(10):701-12.

12. Drossman DA, Chang L, Schneck S, Blackman C, Norton WF, Norton NJ. A focus group assessment of patient perspectives on irritable bowel syndrome and illness severity. *Digestive Diseases and Sciences* 2009;54(7):1532-41.

13. Rønnevig M, Vandvik PO, Bergbom I. Patients' experiences of living with irritable bowel syndrome. *Journal of Advanced Nursing* 2009;65(8):1676-85.

14. Dancey CP, Hutton-Young SA, Moye S, Devins GM. Perceived stigma, illness intrusiveness and quality of life in men and women with irritable bowel syndrome. *Psychology, Health & Medicine* 2002;7(4):381-95.

15. Taft TH, Keefer L, Artz C, Bratten J, Jones MP. Perceptions of illness stigma in patients with inflammatory bowel disease and irritable bowel syndrome. *Quality of Life Research* 2011;20(9):1391-9.

16. Hakanson C, Sahlberg-Blom E, Ternestedt BM. Being in the patient position: experiences of healthcare among people with irritable bowel syndrome. *Qualitative Health Research* 2010;20(8):1116-27.

17. Lackner JM, Brasel AM, Quigley BM, Keefer L, Krasner SS, Powell C, et al. The ties that bind: perceived social support, stress, and IBS in severely affected patients. *Neurogastroenterology & Motility* 2010;22(8):893-900.

18. Heinrichs M, Baumgartner T, Kirschbaum C, Ehlert U. Social support and oxytocin interact to suppress cortisol and subjective responses to psychosocial stress. *Biological Psychiatry* 2003;54(12):1389-98.

19. Goldsmith G, Levin JS. Effect of sleep quality on symptoms of irritable bowel syndrome. *Digestive Diseases and Sciences* 1993;38(10):1809-14.

20. Mearin F, Lacy BE. Diagnostic criteria in IBS: useful or not? *Neurogastroenterology & Motility* 2012;24(9):791-801.

21. Peters HP, De Vries WR, Vanberge-Henegouwen GP, Akkermans LM. Potential benefits and hazards of physical activity and exercise on the gastrointestinal tract. *Gut* 2001;48(3):435-9.

22. De Schryver AM, Keulemans YC, Peters HP, Akkermans LM, Smout

AJ, De Vries WR, et al. Effects of regular physical activity on defecation pattern in middle-aged patients complaining of chronic constipation. *Scandinavian Journal of Gastroenterology* 2005;40(4):422-9.

23. Lustyk MK, Jarrett ME, Bennett JC, Heitkemper MM. Does a physically active lifestyle improve symptoms in women with irritable bowel syndrome? *Gastroenterology Nursing* 2001;24(3):129-37.

24. Hysing M, Pallesen S, Stormark KM, Jakobsen R, Lundervold AJ, Sivertsen B. Sleep and use of electronic devices in adolescence: results from a large population-based study. *BMJ Open* 2015;5(1):e006748.

25. Mullin GE, Shepherd SJ, Chander Roland B, Ireton-Jones C, Matarese LE. Irritable bowel syndrome: contemporary nutrition management strategies. JPEN – *Journal of Parenteral & Enteral Nutrition* 2014;38(7):781-99.

26. Costabile A, Santarelli S, Claus SP, Sanderson J, Hudspith BN, Brostoff J, et al. Effect of breadmaking process on in vitro gut microbiota parameters in irritable bowel syndrome. *PLoS One* 2014;9(10):e111225.

27. Barrett JS. Extending our knowledge of fermentable, short-chain carbohydrates for managing gastrointestinal symptoms. *Nutrition in Clinical Practice* 2013;28(3):300-6.

28. Rogha M, Esfahani MZ, Zargarzadeh AH. The efficacy of a synbiotic containing Bacillus Coagulans in treatment of irritable bowel syndrome: a randomized placebo-controlled trial. *Gastroenterology and Hepatology from Bed to Bench* 2014;7(3):156-63.

29. Tzounis X, Rodriguez-Mateos A, Vulevic J, Gibson GR, Kwik-Uribe C, Spencer JP. Prebiotic evaluation of cocoa-derived flavanols in healthy humans by using a randomized, controlled, double-blind, crossover intervention study. *American Journal of Clinical Nutrition* 2011;93(1):62-72.

30. Brickman AM, Khan UA, Provenzano FA, Yeung LK, Suzuki W, Schroeter H, et al. Enhancing dentate gyrus function with dietary flavanols improves cognition in older adults. *Nature Neuroscience* 2014;17(12):1798-803.

31. Efsa NDAP. Scientific opinion on the substantiation of a health claim related to cocoa flavanols and maintenance of normal endothelium-

dependent vasodilation pursuant to Article 13 (5) of Regulation (EC) No 1924/2006. *European Food Safety Authority Journal* 2012;10(2809):b52.

32. Ford AC, Talley NJ, Spiegel BM, Foxx-Orenstein AE, Schiller L, Quigley EM, et al. Effect of fibre, antispasmodics, and peppermint oil in the treatment of irritable bowel syndrome: systematic review and meta-analysis. *British Medical Journal* 2008;337:a2313.

33. Yoon SL, Grundmann O, Koepp L, Farrell L. Management of irritable bowel syndrome (IBS) in adults: conventional and complementary/ alternative approaches. *Alternative Medicine Review* 2011;16(2):134-51.

34. Whorwell PJ, Prior A, Faragher EB. Controlled trial of hypnotherapy in the treatment of severe refractory irritable bowel syndrome. *Lancet* 1984;2(8414):1232-4.

35. Whorwell PJ, Prior A, Colgan SM. Hypnotherapy in severe irritable bowel syndrome: further experience. *Gut* 1987;28(4):423-5.

36. Palsson OS. Standardized hypnosis treatment for irritable bowel syndrome: the North Carolina protocol. *International Journal of Clinical and Experimental Hypnosis* 2006;54(1):51-64.

37. Greene B, Blanchard EB. Cognitive therapy for irritable bowel syndrome. *Journal of Consulting and Clinical Psychology* 1994;62(3):576-82.

38. Payne A, Blanchard EB. A controlled comparison of cognitive therapy and self-help support groups in the treatment of irritable bowel syndrome. *Journal of Consulting and Clinical Psychology* 1995;63(5):779-86.

39. Lackner JM, Mesmer C, Morley S, Dowzer C, Hamilton S. Psychological treatments for irritable bowel syndrome: a systematic review and meta-analysis. *Journal of Consulting and Clinical Psychology* 2004;72(6):1100-13.

40. Blanchard EB, Lackner JM, Sanders K, Krasner S, Keefer L, Payne A, et al. A controlled evaluation of group cognitive therapy in the treatment of irritable bowel syndrome. *Behaviour Research and Therapy* 2007;45(4):633-48.

41. Bolen BB. Breaking the bonds of irritable bowel syndrome: a psychological approach to regaining control of your life. New Harbinger Publications, Incorporated; 2000.

42. Sanders KA, Blanchard EB, Sykes MA. Preliminary study of a self-administered treatment for irritable bowel syndrome: comparison to a wait list control group. *Applied Psychophysiology and Biofeedback* 2007;32(2):111-9.

43. Davidson RJ, Kabat-Zinn J, Schumacher J, Rosenkranz M, Muller D, Santorelli SF, et al. Alterations in brain and immune function produced by mindfulness meditation. *Psychosomatic Medicine* 2003;65(4):564-70.

44. Gaylord SA, Palsson OS, Garland EL, Faurot KR, Coble RS, Mann JD, et al. Mindfulness training reduces the severity of irritable bowel syndrome in women: results of a randomized controlled trial. *American Journal of Gastroenterology* 2011;106(9):1678-88.

45. Zernicke KA, Campbell TS, Blustein PK, Fung TS, Johnson JA, Bacon SL, et al. Mindfulness-based stress reduction for the treatment of irritable bowel syndrome symptoms: a randomized wait-list controlled trial. *International Journal of Behavioral Medicine* 2013;20(3):385-96.

46. Ljøtsson B, Andreewitch S, Hedman E, Ruck C, Andersson G, Lindefors N. Exposure and mindfulness-based therapy for irritable bowel syndrome – an open pilot study. *Journal of Behavior Therapy and Experimental Psychiatry* 2010;41(3):185-90.

47. Ljøtsson B, Falk L, Vesterlund AW, Hedman E, Lindfors P, Ruck C, et al. Internet-delivered exposure and mindfulness-based therapy for irritable bowel syndrome – a randomized controlled trial. *Behaviour Research and Therapy* 2010;48(6):531-9.

48. Coulson NS. Receiving social support online: an analysis of a computer-mediated support group for individuals living with irritable bowel syndrome. *Cyberpsychology and Behavior* 2005;8(6):580-4.

49. Wainwright M, Russell AJ, Yiannakou Y. Challenging the biopsychosocial model in a chronic constipation clinic. *Qualitative Health Research* 2011;21(12):1643-57.

50. Casiday RE, Hungin AP, Cornford CS, de Wit NJ, Blell MT. GPs' explanatory models for irritable bowel syndrome: a mismatch with patient models? *Family Practice* 2009;26(1):34-9.

51. Harkness EF, Harrington V, Hinder S, O'Brien SJ, Thompson DG, Beech

P, et al. GP perspectives of irritable bowel syndrome – an accepted illness, but management deviates from guidelines: a qualitative study. *Family Practice* 2013;14:92.

52. Casiday RE, Hungin AP, Cornford CS, de Wit NJ, Blell MT. Patients' explanatory models for irritable bowel syndrome: symptoms and treatment more important than explaining aetiology. *Family Practice* 2009;26(1):40-7.

53. Bengtson MB, Ronning T, Vatn MH, Harris JR. Irritable bowel syndrome in twins: genes and environment. *Gut* 2006;55(12):1754-9.

54. Saito YA. The role of genetics in IBS. *Gastroenterology Clinics of North America* 2011;40(1):45-67.

55. Drossman DA, Grant Thompson W, Talley NJ, Funch-Jensen P, Janssens J, Whitehead WE. Identification of subgroups of functional gastrointestinal disorder. *Gastroenterology International* 1990;3(4):159-72.

56. Neal KR, Hebden J, Spiller R. Prevalence of gastrointestinal symptoms six months after bacterial gastroenteritis and risk factors for development of the irritable bowel syndrome: postal survey of patients. *British Medical Journal* 1997;314(7083):779-82.

57. Vermeire S, Van Assche G, Rutgeerts P. Postinfectious irritable bowel syndrome: a genetic link identified? *Gastroenterology* 2010;138:1246–9.

58. Mearin F, Perez-Oliveras M, Perello A, Vinyet J, Ibanez A, Coderch J, et al. Dyspepsia and irritable bowel syndrome after a Salmonella gastroenteritis outbreak: one-year follow-up cohort study *Gastroenterology* 2005;129(1):98-104.

59. Malinen E, Rinttila T, Kajander K, Matto J, Kassinen A, Krogius L, et al. Analysis of the fecal microbiota of irritable bowel syndrome patients and healthy controls with real-time PCR. *American Journal of Gastroenterology* 2005;100(2):373-82.

60. Panda S, El Khader I, Casellas F, Lopez Vivancos J, Garcia Cors M, Santiago A, et al. Short-term effect of antibiotics on human gut microbiota. *PLoS One* 2014;9(4):e95476.

61. Rhee SH, Pothoulakis C, Mayer EA. Principles and clinical

implications of the brain–gut–enteric microbiota axis. *Nature Reviews Gastroenterology and Hepatology* 2009;6(5):306-14.

62. Klooker TK, Braak B, Painter RC, de Rooij SR, van Elburg RM, van den Wijngaard RM, et al. Exposure to severe wartime conditions in early life is associated with an increased risk of irritable bowel syndrome: a population-based cohort study. *American Journal of Gastroenterology* 2009;104(9):2250-6.

63. Lackner JM, Gudleski GD, Blanchard EB. Beyond abuse: the association among parenting style, abdominal pain, and somatization in IBS patients. *Behaviour Research and Therapy* 2004;42(1):41-56.

64. Collins SM, Bercik P. The relationship between intestinal microbiota and the central nervous system in normal gastrointestinal function and disease. *Gastroenterology* 2009;136(6):2003-14.

65. Zhou Q, Zhang B, Verne GN. Intestinal membrane permeability and hypersensitivity in the irritable bowel syndrome. *Pain* 2009;146(1-2):41-6.

66. Soderholm JD, Yates DA, Gareau MG, Yang PC, MacQueen G, Perdue MH. Neonatal maternal separation predisposes adult rats to colonic barrier dysfunction in response to mild stress. *American Journal of Physiology: Gastrointestinal and Liver Physiology* 2002;283(6):G1257-63.

67. Santos J, Yang PC, Soderholm JD, Benjamin M, Perdue MH. Role of mast cells in chronic stress induced colonic epithelial barrier dysfunction in the rat. *Gut* 2001;48(5):630-6.

68. Barbara G, Stanghellini V, De Giorgio R, Cremon C, Cottrell GS, Santini D, et al. Activated mast cells in proximity to colonic nerves correlate with abdominal pain in irritable bowel syndrome. *Gastroenterology* 2004;126(3):693-702.

69. Chadwick VS, Chen W, Shu D, Paulus B, Bethwaite P, Tie A, et al. Activation of the mucosal immune system in irritable bowel syndrome. *Gastroenterology* 2002;122(7):1778-83.

70. Coates MD, Mahoney CR, Linden DR, Sampson JE, Chen J, Blaszyk H, et al. Molecular defects in mucosal serotonin content and decreased serotonin reuptake transporter in ulcerative colitis and irritable bowel syndrome. *Gastroenterology* 2004;126(7):1657-64.

Appendix

Useful Addresses

The IBS Network
Unit 1.12 SOAR Works
14 Knutton Road
Sheffield S5 9NU, UK
Tel: +44 (0)1142723253
Email: info@theibsnetwork.org
Website: http://www.theibsnetwork.org

Bladder and Bowel Foundation
SATRA Innovation Park
Rockingham Road
Kettering
Northants NN16 9JH, UK
Helpline: +44 (0)845 345 0165
General enquiries: +44 (0)1536 533255
Email: info@bladderandbowelfoundation.org
Website: http://www.bladderandbowelfoundation.org

The British Acupuncture Council
63 Jeddo Road
London W12 9HQ, UK
Tel: +44 (0)20 8735 0400
Fax: +44 (0)20 8735 0404
Email: Via website at (http://www.acupuncture.org.uk/The-British-Acupuncture-Council.html)
Website: www.acupuncture.org.uk

The Hypnotherapy Association UK
14 Crown Street
Chorley
Lancashire PR7 1DX, UK
Tel: +44 (0)1257 262124
Email: b.h.a@btconnect.com
Website: www.thehypnotherapyassociation.co.uk

The National Hypnotherapy Society
PO Box 131
Arundel
West Sussex BN18 8BR, UK
Tel: +44 (0)870 850 3387
Email: admin@nationalhypnotherapysociety.org
Website: www.nationalhypnotherapysociety.org

The General Hypnotherapy Standards Council (GHSC) and General Hypnotherapy Register (GHR)
PO Box 204
Lymington SO41 6WP, UK
Email: admin@general-hypnotherapy-register.com
Website: www.general-hypnotherapy-register.com

Complementary and Natural Healthcare Council
83 Victoria Street
London SW1H 0HW, UK
Tel: +44 (0)20 3178 2199 between 9.30 a.m. and 5.30 p.m.,
Monday to Friday
Email: info@cnhc.org.uk
Website: www.cnhc.org.uk

Index

Managing IBD
A balanced guide to Inflammatory Bowel Disease

By Jenna Farmer
with Kay Greveson RGN MSc and Sally Baker

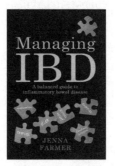

Jenna Farmer offers an holistic and positive guide to living with IBD, combining conventional medical knowledge, nutrition tips, stress reduction advice and other lifestyle approaches, drawing on her blog posts, ebooks and website www.abalancedbelly.co.uk. Throughout, the book features case histories from Jenna's blog and other contacts, and from her own experience of delayed diagnosis and listening to her symptoms. And Jenna calls on health professionals Kay Greveson (specialist IBD nurse and founder of IBDPassport) and Sally Baker (therapist specialising in anxiety, stress and emotional eating) for their expert guidance.

Sustainable Medicine
Whistle-blowing on 21st century medical practice

By Dr Sarah Myhill

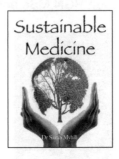

Suppressing symptoms with drugs and then suppressing the side effects of those drugs with yet more drugs is not a sustainable model for good health. In *Sustainable Medicine*, Dr Myhill shows the importance of identifying the root cause of any symptoms we may have, how we can do that, and what we can do to keep ourselves healthy and resilient.

The most important things we must do are to reduce any inflammation in our bodies, largely through an anti-inflammatory diet, and build our immunity so that we can withstand potential infection. *Sustainable Medicine* is the self-help guide to understanding and achieving those goals.

'This book is an invitation for patients and practitioners alike to move away from a culture of ignorance, restrictive guidelines and blame and to make informed decisions and take responsibility for their own health again.'

Dr Franziska Meuschel MD, PhD, ND, LFhom

www.hammersmithbooks.co.uk/ product/sustainable-medicine/

Nature Cures
The A to Z of Ailments and Natural Foods

By Nat H Hawes

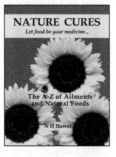

Nearly 2500 year ago, Hippocrates, the 'father of medicine', recognised the importance to human health of what is consumed as food and drink. While research in the intervening time has continually supported this, and knowledge of nutrients and their relationship to health has galloped forward in recent years, as part of everyday life, the age-old wisdom of health benefits and healing properties of natural unprocessed foods has dwindled away and now, when health becomes compromised, our first reaction is to head for the medicine cabinet or the doctor.

Nature Cures redresses our missing knowledge by bringing together a vast compendium of traditional wisdom, contemporary specialist knowledge and the latest research findings, organised in a way that makes it easy to find the food, nutrient or ailment that is relevant whenever required.

Let food truly be your medicine, and medicine your food...

www.hammersmithbooks.co.uk/product/nature-cures/

What's Up With Your Gut?
Why you bloat after eating bread and pasta...
and other gut problems

By Jo Waters and Professor Julian Walters

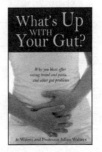

Do you get bloating when you eat pasta? Is your social life restricted by uncertainty about your bowels? Is your ability to work affected? This book will help you find out what your underlying gut problem is and understand how to make things better. With 80% of our immune system in our gut, sorting out digestive problems is essential for good health.

What's Up With Your Gut? takes a practical look at the full range of gut problems, using a symptom-led approach so that sufferers can recognise what may have been troubling them for years and find solutions.
It then describes the range of solutions, both standard and alternative, emphasising the importance of what is eaten/food intolerances and the impact of poor digestion on overall health. Whether you suffer cramping diarrhoea when you are stressed out, get constipated when you're on holiday or just feel fatigued by your grumbling guts, they show what the options are for diagnosis, symptom improvement and tackling the underlying causes.

www.hammersmithbooks.co.uk/product/your-gut/